Pediatric Nurse Practitioner Certification Study Question Book

EDITOR

Virginia Layng Millonig, Ph.D., R.N., C.P.N.P.
President
Health Leadership Associates, Inc.
Potomac, Maryland

Health Leadership Associates
Potomac, Maryland

Question Books

Family Nurse Practitioner Certification Study Question Set

(ISBN 1-878028-26-X)

by
Health Leadership Associates, Inc.

Consists of

The

Adult Nurse Practitioner Certification Study Question Book
ISBN 1-878028-20-0

Pediatric Nurse Practitioner Certification Study Question Book
ISBN 1-878028-21-9

Women's Health Nurse Practitioner Certification Study Question Book
ISBN 1-878028-22-7

Additional Nursing Certification Study Question Books by Health Leadership Associates, Inc.

Acute Care Nurse Practitioner Certification Study Question Book
(ISBN# 1-878028-25-1), List Price $30.00

Adult Nurse Practitioner Certification Study Question Book
(ISBN# 1-878028-20-0), List Price $30.00

Pediatric Nurse Practitioner Certification Study Question Book
(ISBN# 1-878028-21-9), List Price $30.00

Women's Health Nurse Practitioner Certification Study Question Book
(ISBN# 1-878028-22-7), List Price $30.00

Family Nurse Practitioner Certification Study Question Book Set
(This shrink wrapped set consists of the Adult, Pediatric, and Women's Health Study Question Books).
(ISBN# 1-878028-26-X). List Price $60.00

Certification Review Books

Family Nurse Practitioner Set

(ISBN 1-878028-24-3)

by
Health Leadership Associates, Inc.

Consists of
The

**Adult Nurse Practitioner Certification
Review Guide
(3rd edition)**

**Pediatric Nurse Practitioner Certification
Review Guide
(3rd edition)**

**Women's Health Care Nurse Practitioner
Certification Review Guide**

Health Leadership Associates, Inc.
Managing Editor: Mary A. Millonig
Production Manager: Martha M. Pounsberry
Editorial Assistants: Bridget M. Jones
                        Cheryl C. Patterson
Cover and Design: Merrifield Graphics
Composition: Port City Press, Inc.
Design and Production: Port City Press, Inc.

Printed in the United States of America

Health Leadership Associates, Inc.
P.O. Box 59153
Potomac, Maryland 20859

Library of Congress Cataloging-in-Publication Data

Pediatric nurse practitioner certification study question book /
   editor, Virginia Layng Millonig.
        p. cm. — (Family nurse practitioner certification study
question set)
   Includes bibliographical references.
   ISBN 1-878028-21-9 (paperback). — ISBN 1-878028-26-X (set)
   1. Pediatric nursing—Examinations Study guides.   2. Nurse
practitioners—Examinations Study guides.   I. Millonig, Virginia
Layng.   II. Series.
   [DNLM: 1. Nurse Practitioners Examination Questions.   2. Pediatric
Nursing—methods Examination Questions.   WY 18.2 P3712 1999]
RJ245.P394   1999
610.73'62'076—dc21
DNLM/DLC
for Library of Congress   99-22759
                                                             CIP

10 9 8 7 6 5 4 3 2
Second printing March 1999

Contributing Authors

Patricia K. Clinton, Ph.D., R.N., C.P.N.P.
Pediatric Nurse Practitioner
Clinical Assistant Professor
Director, Pediatric Nurse Practitioner Program
College of Nursing
The University of Iowa
Iowa City, Iowa

Brenda Holloway, M.S.N., R.N.,C.S., F.N.P.
Family Nurse Practitioner
Assistant Clinical Professor
University of South Alabama
Mobile, Alabama

Martha K. Swartz, M.S., R.N.,C.S., P.N.P.
Pediatric Nurse Practitioner
Associate Professor
Pediatric Nurse Practitioner Program
Yale University School of Nursing
Pediatric Nurse Practitioner
Yale New Haven Hospital
New Haven, Connecticut

Reviewers

Teri M. Woo, M.S., R.N., C.P.N.P.
Pediatric Nurse Practitioner
Adjunct Faculty
Child and Family Nursing
College of Nursing
Oregon Health Sciences University
Portland, Oregon

Ruth G. Mullins, Ph.D.(c)., R.N., C.P.N.P.
Pediatric Nurse Practitioner
Professor
Department of Nursing
California State University, Long Beach
Long Beach, California

Preface

Health Leadership Associates is pleased to introduce one more component to our complement of Nurse Practitioner Certification Review materials. This "Pediatric Nurse Practitioner Certification Study Question Book" will further assist the user of this book to be successful in the examination process. It should by no means be the only source used for preparation for the Pediatric or Family Nurse Practitioner Certification examinations. It has been developed primarily to enhance your test taking skills while also integrating the principles (becoming test-wise) of test taking found in the "Test Taking Strategies and Skills" chapter of the "Pediatric Nurse Practitioner Certification Review Guide" published by Health Leadership Associates. This review guide in addition to the review courses and home study programs provides a comprehensive and total approach to success in the examination process. It enables the users of these materials to be successful in the test taking process, and reinforces the knowledge base that is critical in the delivery of care in the practice setting. Many individuals feel that taking practice test questions is the most important factor in the certification examination preparation process, yet it is but one strategy to be used in combination with a strong knowledge base. Success in the certification examination area is based upon both excellent test taking skills and a comprehensive understanding of the content of the examination. As a nurse practitioner seeking certification, it is important to not lose sight of the definition and purpose of certification. "Certification is a process by which nongovernmental agencies or associations confirm that an individual licensed to practice as a professional has met certain predetermined standards specified by that profession for specialty practice." Its purpose is to assure the public that an individual has mastered a body of knowledge and acquired skills in a particular specialty" (ANA, 1979).

Inherent to the preparation for certification examinations is rigorous attention to the directives and materials from the certification boards. Content outlines and sample test questions are often provided to examinees prior to the examinations. Specifics for each examination including suggested readings will be provided by the individual testing boards.

This question book has been prepared by board certified nurse practitioners. The questions have then been reviewed and critiqued by board certified nurse practitioners (content experts) and a test construction specialist. There are 300 problem oriented certification board-type multiple choice questions which are divided according to content area (based upon testing board content outlines) with answers, rationales and a reference list. Every effort has been made to develop sample questions that are representative of the types of questions that may be found on the certification examinations, however, style and format of the examination may differ. Engaging in the exercise of test taking, an understanding of test taking strategies, and knowledge in respective content areas can only lead to success.

CONTENTS

Growth and Development

Patricia Clinton

Select one best answer to the following questions.

1. H.O. is a 5-year-old Vietnamese child who has fallen off of his growth curve. The best intervention would be to:

    a. Suggest infant breakfast drinks as supplements
    b. Incorporate traditional foods into a management plan
    c. Educate the family on need for increased calories and nutrients
    c. Refer family to growth clinic for evaluation

2. While taking the history of 6-month-old E.M. you learn that she is not sleeping through the night, and will not fall back to sleep without the parents rocking or feeding her. This is an example of:

    a. Somnambulism
    b. Pavor nocturnus
    c. Learned behavior
    d. Delayed sleep phase

3. Which of the following scenarios is suggestive of a child who may not be ready to enter first grade? The ability to:

    a. Recognize six colors and remember his phone number
    b. Use scissors and follow three step directions
    c. Name best friend and hold crayons appropriately
    d. Count to five and draw a person with three parts

4. T.T. is a 9-week-old preterm infant whose birth weight was 2.3 kg. Mom was HB_s Ag negative. He is seen today for the first time since discharge from the nursery. The appropriate immunizations to give at this time would be:

    a. DTaP, Hib, IPV, Hep B-1
    b. DTP, Hib, OPV, Hep B-1

    c. DTaP, Hib, IPV
- d. DTaP, Hib, OPV

5. While examining 10-year-old R.M.'s teeth you note that the upper incisors slightly overlap the lower incisors. The second and lower first molars are absent. Your assessment is:

    a. Malocclusion
- b. Delayed mandibular dentition
    c. Normal dentition
    d. Hyperdontia

6. The mother of 5-year-old D.W. is concerned that her son often cheats when playing board games with his older sister. What is the most appropriate response to D.W.'s behavior?

    a. Encourage the parent to use five minute time-outs when cheating occurs
- b. Explain that developmentally D.W. is unable to comprehend rigid rules
    c. Suggest that until D.W. is older he should not play board games with his sibling
    d. Explain to D.W. that cheating is like lying and is not acceptable behavior

7. Which of the following is not a sign of readiness to toilet train?

    a. Can sit for extended periods
    b. Can follow directions
    c. Occasional waking from naps with dry diapers
    d. Regularity of bowel movements

8. Which of the following physical findings in a 2-month-old child warrants an immediate referral to a physician?

    a. Head circumference growing faster than height and weight
    b. Overriding lambdoidal sutures
    c. Rigid and immobile sagittal suture
    d. Snapping sensation when pressure applied to parietal bone

9. While listening to 2½-year-old K.L. talk, you note that she frequently omits final consonants and her sentences are 2 to 3 words in length. The appropriate plan of care would be:

    a. Routine follow-up at next well child visit
    b. Referring for hearing screen
    c. Assessing for developmental delays

    d. Referring to a speech pathologist

10. The mother of 3-year-old G.W. reports that he has begun to stutter. Further probing reveals that the stuttering occurs frequently and lasts 1 to 2 seconds. G.W. does not seem bothered by the stuttering. The appropriate management would be:

    a. Referral to a speech pathologist
    b. Re-evaluation in one year
    c. Reassuring mom that this is a mild problem
    d. To demonstrate to G.W. slow, deep breathing before talking

11. You would expect a school age child to:

    a. Grow $1\frac{1}{2}$ inches per year
    b. Grow $\frac{1}{2}$ inch per year
    c. Gain about 6 pounds per year
    d. Gain about 3 pounds per year

12. During 8-month-old L.B.'s physical examination, dad boasts that he is going to be a left handed batter since he prefers doing everything with his left hand. The appropriate response would be to:

    a. Ask if others in the family are left handed
    b. Suggest play activities that require using both hands
    c. Present toys more often to the right hand
    d. Perform a careful neurological examination

13. 12-year-old Peter has been diagnosed with constitutional growth delay. Appropriate management would include:

    a. Starting low dose testosterone therapy now
    b. Counseling regarding delayed onset of puberty
    c. Thyroxine replacement
    d. Nutritional counseling

14. Which of the following best describes behavior associated with Piaget's concrete operations?

    a. Learning primarily by trial and error
    b. Interpreting events in relationship to themselves
    c. Categorizing information into lower to higher classes
    d. Drawing logical conclusions from observations

15. 8-year-old Jeffrey has been diagnosed with ADHD. In addition to medication, which of the following nutritional interventions would be least helpful?

    a. Monthly height and weight checks
    b. Small frequent meals and snacks
    c. High calorie supplemental drinks
    d. Elimination of refined sugar from diet

16. The principle that growth and development becomes increasingly integrated is best demonstrated by:

    a. Gaining head control before raising the chest
    b. Bringing cup to mouth, tipping, and swallowing
    c. Rolling over before sitting
    d. Grasping with fist before using fingers

17. In males, Tanner Stage III can be distinguished from Tanner Stage II by:

    a. Fine, downy pubic hair at the base of penis
    b. Adult like pubic hair not extending to thighs
    c. Penile growth in width
    d. Penile growth in length

18. 13-year-old T.J. reluctantly shares with you that his "chest hurts." On physical examination you note unilateral breast enlargement which is tender to palpation. You suspect physiological gynecomastia. Which Tanner stage would support that diagnosis?

    a. Tanner stage I
    b. Tanner stage III
    c. Tanner stage IV
    d. Tanner stage V

19. During a physical examination of 10½-year-old Melissa you note the appearance of breast buds. You tell her that she can expect which of the following in approximately 2 years?

    a. Growth of pubic hair
    b. Peak height velocity
    c. Onset of menses
    d. Axillary hair

20. Adolescents who engage in risky behavior, such as driving without a seat belt, are displaying:

a. A type of egocentrism
b. A need for independence
c. Role experimentation
d. Low self-esteem

21. An increase in which of the following behaviors is seen more frequently in late, rather than early, adolescence?

a. Value conflict with parents
b. Focus on physical appearance
c. Peer group involvement
d. Understanding inner motivations of others

Answers and Rationale

1. **(b)** It is important for health care professionals to understand the cultural norms and perspectives of others. This often helps in compliance with suggestions for improved health. Asian families, out of respect, do not often ask questions or challenge advice. By understanding their food patterns, and incorporating that into a diet plan, compliance may increase (Burns, et al., p. 61).

2. **(c)** Sleepwalking (somnabulism) and pavor nocturnus (night terrors) are sleep disturbances which occur in school age and preschool age children respectively. Learned behavior is a result of parents interfering with the child's attempts to return to sleep without stimulation from the parents (Burns, et al., p. 319).

3. **(d)** Children entering first grade should have the requisite skills to master the tasks they will encounter. This includes language, fine and gross motor skills, and personal and social skills. At this age the child should be able to draw a person with at least 6 parts and count to 10 or more (Fox, pp. 263-269; Burns, et al., pp. 133).

4. **(a)** Preterm infants should be immunized at the usual chronologic age with the regular doses. IPV should be given to avoid nosocomial transmission of polio virus vaccine strain (AAP, p. 48).

5. **(b)** The mandibular (lower) molars usually erupt between ages 6 to 7. Even allowing for individual variation, this is a considerable delay. Hyperdontia refers to supernumerary teeth (Burns, et al., p. 683; Zitelli & Davis, p. 610).

6. **(b)** Developmentally, the concept of cheating is not well understood until the age of 7 years. The idea of playing fairly to ensure everyone an equal chance occurs with maturity and the ability to differentiate among moral choices (Fox, p. 287).

7. **(d)** Regularity of bowel movements is established early in infancy but has nothing to do with voluntary sphincter control necessary for toilet training (Burns, et al., pp. 277-280).

8. **(c)** Ridged and immobile sutures indicates premature fusing resulting in cranio-synostosis. For proper brain growth, sutures need to approximate each other yet remain mobile (Fox, p. 682).

9. **(a)** 2 to 3 year olds have several articulation dysfluencies, among them the dropping of final consonants. 2 to 3 word sentences are normal for the 24 to 30 month old child (Burns, et al., pp. 108-110).

10. **(c)** This represents a mild stuttering problem but does not warrant immediate referral unless the child or parent are increasingly concerned, or if it continues indefinitely (Hoekelman, et al., p. 755).

11. **(c)** The recognized standard of physical growth of school age children is to gain 5 to 7 pounds per year and grow about 2.5 inches per year (Burns, et al., p. 125).

12. **(d)** Handedness before a year is cause for concern and may indicate cerebral palsy. A neurological examination is indicated. The examiner should carefully assess for increase in deep tendon reflexes and tone (Burns, et al., pp. 103, 558).

13. **(b)** Constitutional growth delay is considered a variant of normal, marked by delayed onset of puberty. Final growth is achieved later but is consistent with family genetics. Growth hormone or thyroxine is not recommended. Nutritional therapies will not change the outcome. Low dose hormone therapy is appropriate for selected individuals with psychosocial concerns beginning at age 14 (Burns, et al., p. 522; Behrman, et al., p. 653).

14. **(c)** Concrete operations occur during the school age years as children begin to understand the characteristics of things and objects. Classification is a thought process that develops during this time (Burns, et al., p. 125).

15. **(d)** Stimulant medication may decrease the appetite so careful monitoring of growth and a nutritional plan that encourages adequate calories is important. There is no sound evidence that sugar or artificial additives play a role in ADHD (Burns, et al., p. 332; Hoekelman, et al., p. 678).

16. **(b)** Infants must first develop hand-mouth coordination before incorporating tipping and swallowing, which is a more integrated function. Head control before raising the chest demonstrates the principle of cephalocaudal progression. Options "c" and "d" suggest proximal-distal progression (Burns, et al., p. 68).

17. **(d)** Most penile growth in Tanner Stage III is in length rather than width due to underdevelopment of the corpora cavernosa. Fine downy pubic hair appears in Stage II and adult like appearance occurs in Stage IV (Burns, et al., p. 145).

18. **(b)** Physiologic gynecomastia is a common clinical finding in young adolescent males. It is usually present during Tanner Stage III (Behrman, et al., p. 235).

19. **(c)** Understanding the sequencing of pubertal development is important, but it must be remembered that individual timing may differ. In the female patient, pubic hair, axillary hair, and the peak height velocity generally occur before menarche (Burns, et al., p. 143-145).

20. **(a)** The belief that one is immune from poor or bad outcomes (e.g., death, disease) is a form of egocentrism known as personal fable in which adolescents believes that the laws of nature do not apply to them (Burns, et al., p. 148; Behrman, et al., pp. 16, 232).

21. **(d)** Late adolescence is characterized by increased autonomy and a beginning appreciation of the complexities and motivations of other's behaviors (Burns, et al., pp. 152-153).

References

American Academy of Pediatrics (AAP). (1997). *Redbook: Report of the committee on infectious diseases* (24th ed.). Elk Grove Village, IL: Author.

Behrman, R. E., & Kliegman, R. M. (Eds.). (1998). *Nelson essentials of pediatrics* (3rd ed.). Philadelphia: W. B. Saunders.

Burns, C. E., Barber, N., Brady, M. A., & Dunn, A. M. (Eds.). (1997). *Pediatric primary care: A handbook for nurse practitioners.* Philadelphia: W. B. Saunders.

Fox, J. A. (Ed.). (1997). *Primary health care of children.* St. Louis: Mosby.

Hoekelman, R. A., Friedman, S. B., Nelson, N. M., Seidel, H. M., & Weitzman, M. L. (Eds.). (1997). *Primary pediatric care.* St. Louis: Mosby.

Zitelli, B. J., & Davis, H. W. (Eds.). (1997). *Atlas of pediatric physical diagnosis* (3rd ed.). St. Louis: Mosby.

Note: This chapter was written by Patricia Clinton prior to her appointment as certification chair representing the National Association of Pediatric Nurse Associates and Practitioners (NAPNAP) to the National Certification Board of Pediatric Nurse Practitioners and Nurses.

Health Promotion and Maintenance

Martha K. Swartz

Select one best answer to the following questions.

1. You detect a heart murmur while examining a 3-year-old child. In determining whether or not a referral is necessary, you recall that "innocent" heart murmurs are associated with which of the following signs?

    a. Best heard during diastole
    b. Radiation to the axilla
    c. Intensity is no greater than I or II/VI
    d. No variation with change in child's position

2. When providing anticipatory guidance about infant development, you may teach parents that a normal infant may first transfer an object from hand to hand at:

    a. 2 months of age
    b. 4 months of age
    c. 7 months of age
    d. 9 months of age

3. A 2-month-old infant at your clinic received a combined DPT/Hib vaccine and the parents are in need of teaching about possible side effects. Which of the following is not an adverse effect following administration of the whole-cell DPT vaccination:

    a. Local reaction
    b. Fever
    c. Increased fussiness
    d. Transient morbilliform rash (mmR)

4. When reviewing immunization protocols at your clinic, you are aware that the varicella zoster virus vaccine can be administered to susceptible children beginning at what age?

    a. 4 months
    b. 6 months
  — c. 12 months
    d. 15 months

5. A 3-week-old is in the clinic for a scheduled weight check. The best indication that a 3-week-old infant is ingesting sufficient breast milk is that the baby:

  — a. Passes at least four stools per day
    b. Feeds every three hours
    c. Voids five times a day
    d. Has lost no more than 10% of its birthweight

6. A mother of an 8-month-old infant asks you for advice about continued intro-duction of solids. You recommend which of the following food groups be intro-duced to the baby last?

    a. Egg yolk
  — b. Egg white — *protein allergy risk*
    c. Fruits
    d. Vegetables

7. The mother of a 15-month-old infant informs you that she feeds the baby skim milk. You advise the mother to change to whole milk primarily because skim milk:

    a. Is not as easily digested as whole milk
    b. Contains an insufficient amount of calcium
    c. Contains too little protein
  — d. Provides an inadequate amount of essential fatty acids

8. An adolescent is being evaluated for childhood depression. Which behavior or sign is least likely to be evident?

  — a. Evidence of hallucinations and delusions
    b. A history of recurrent "accidents"
    c. A sense of guilt
    d. The presence of eating disorders

9. A 12-year-old boy is brought into the clinic for an urgent visit after having in-gested 10 diazepam tablets. Following the initial emergent care and stabiliza-tion of the child, the most important aspect of your management is:

    a. Referring the case to the child welfare department

b. Assessing the family supports available to the child
— c. Obtaining a psychiatric consultation
d. Reviewing the history for signs of depression

10. You are seeing a 15-month-old boy with documented human immunodeficiency virus (HIV) infection for a check-up. If indicated, this child may receive all of the following vaccines except:

a. Measles, mumps, and rubella (MMR)
b. *H. influenzae* type B (Hib)
c. Diphtheria, tetanus, acellular pertussis (DTaP)
— d. Oral poliovirus vaccine (OPV)

11. While conducting the Denver II developmental screening test, the mother of an 18-month-old child reports to you that the toddler does not imitate activities. You decide to assess the child's development further by giving him tasks from what sector:

— a. Personal-social *to R/O autism*
b. Fine motor-adaptive
c. Language
d. Gross motor

12. You have ordered routine blood screening for a 2-year-old girl who, because of dietary habits, is at risk for iron deficiency anemia. Which of the following findings is not associated with iron deficiency anemia?

a. Hypochromic RBC   *IDA — hypochromic*
b. Microcytic RBC   *microcytic*
c. Low reticulocyte count   *↑FEP*
↑RDW ↓mcv
— d. Low free erythrocyte protoporphyrin (FEP) level   *IDA assoc c̄ ↑FEP*

13. During a prenatal visit, you review the mother's record for routine prenatal screening results. While educating the mother, you explain that the maternal serum screening of alpha-fetoprotein (AFP) between the 15th and 21st weeks of pregnancy is done primarily to screen for:

a. Phenylketonuria
b. Galactosemia
c. Cystic fibrosis
— d. Neural tube defects

14. A tenderness is detected over the tibial tuberosity of a 10-year-old boy during a

routine examination at a school based clinic. The PNP knows this may be a sign of:

- — a. Osgood-Schlatter disease
- b. Blount's disease
- c. Plantar fasciitis
- d. Effusion in the joint space

15. The parents of a 1-week-old infant are concerned about the unusual shape of their child's head. In the physical examination of this infant, which of the following signs would not support a diagnosis of craniosynostosis?

- a. Palpation of a ridge along a given suture line
- b. Unusual skull configuration
- — c. A palpable lesion at the occipital region
- d. Abnormal head circumference

16. In the emergency room, you encounter a toddler whose injuries are not consistent with the history that is given. Which of the following would be the best step a provider could take in order to foster communication with abusive parents?

- a. Realize that abusive parents have essentially different goals for their children than do other caregivers
- — b. Understand that parental hostility and resistance are potent symptoms of fear and inadequacy
- c. Consider referring the parent to a substance abuse program
- d. Be cautious when sharing the results of medical findings

17. You are preparing a drug prevention program for middle school students. Your educational approach is based on the knowledge that the most common substance of abuse in adolescence is:

- a. Marijuana
- b. Cocaine
- c. Heroin
- — d. Alcohol

18. During a check-up of a 15-month-old girl, you note that the child has dropped significantly in percentile for weight over the past few months. In evaluating a child with failure to thrive, the most important part of your assessment involves:

- — a. The history

b. The physical examination
c. Laboratory studies
d. Observation of family interactions

19. A 7-year-old child in your caseload has recently been placed on methylpheni-
date for behavioral concerns associated with ADHD. Which of the following
side effects are not associated with this drug?

    a. Decreased appetite
    b. Weight loss
    c. Irritability
    — d. Decreased heart rate   *actually, ↑ HR and/or ↑ BP*

20. The parents of an 8-year-old are concerned that their son does not want to at-
tend school. Which of the following historical findings are not usually associated with the diagnosis of school phobia?

    a. Sporadic school absence
    — b. Chronic medical illness
    c. Vague physical symptoms
    d. Depression and anxiety

21. A 17-year-old girl is referred to your clinic by the school nurse to be assessed
for an eating disorder. Which of the following dynamics is not characteristic of
anorexia nervosa?

    — a. Excessive eating followed by purging *— bulimia*
    b. A pervasive sense of helplessness and ineffectiveness
    c. Weight loss gives the patient a sense of mastery and control
    d. Low body temperature, pulse rate, and blood pressure

Answers & Rationale

1. **(c)** Innocent murmurs usually have an intensity of no greater than I or II/VI, occur early in systole, are not likely to radiate over parts of the chest, and the presence and intensity vary with change in the child's position (Grundy, p. 82).

2. **(c)** A normal infant transfers objects from hand to hand by seven months (Grundy, p. 96).

3. **(d)** A transient morbilliform rash is an adverse effect associated with the MMR vaccine (Simoes & Groothuis, p. 245).

4. **(c)** According to the recommended Childhood Immunization Schedule approved by the ACIP and AAP, the varicella vaccine can be administered at 12 months (Simoes & Groothuis, p. 239).

5. **(a)** Breast fed infants under one month of age should be having four or more stools in a 24 hour period. Fewer than four, even if wetting frequently, is considered a danger sign (Eiger, p. 175).

6. **(b)** Rice cereal, the least allergenic of cereals, should be offered first followed by fruits and vegetables, meats, egg yolk and egg white (Eiger, p. 180).

7. **(d)** All milk (human and cow) is deficient in iron. Skim milk should be avoided until age two because it provides too few calories, an excess of protein and an inadequate amount of essential fatty acids (Eiger, p. 179).

8. **(a)** Hallucinations and delusions are uncommon in the presentation of adolescent depression (Hodas, 1997a, p. 920).

9. **(c)** Every actively suicidal patient, regardless of apparent seriousness, requires psychiatric consultation and, in some cases, hospitalization (Hodas, 1997a, p. 920).

10. **(d)** Congenitally immunodeficient children should not be immunized with live-virus or live bacteria vaccines with the exception of the MMR (Simoes & Groothuis, p. 235).

11. **(a)** Imitating activities is considered to be a personal-social task (Simeonsson & Simeonsson, p. 240).

12. **(d)** Iron deficiency anemia is a microcytic, hypochromic anemia associated with a low reticulocyte count and elevated FEP level (Poncz, p. 589).

13. **(d)** The AFP is used primarily to screen for neural tube defects. The other diseases are usually screened for at birth (Holtzman & Braverman, p. 215).

14. **(a)** Tenderness over the tibial tubercle may be a sign of Osgood-Schlatter disease. Blount's disease is characterized by severe bowing of the legs, and plantar fasciitis is associated with painful heels (Grundy, p. 91).

15. **(c)** Diagnosis of craniosynostosis is suspected as a result of skull configuration, a ridge along a suture line, and abnormal head circumference. Other palpable lesions, which often occur in the occipital region, are not indicative of craniosynostosis (Curry, p. 47).

16. **(b)** Parental fear and inadequacy may be manifested as hostility. Abusive parents generally have similar goals for their children as others and are not any more likely to be substance abusers than nonabusive parents. Medical findings should be shared with the parents (without necessarily promoting an etiologic conclusion) (Seidl, pp. 976-979).

17. **(d)** Alcohol is the most common substance of abuse consumed by teenagers (Sargent, 1997a, p. 928).

18. **(a)** The two major causes of poor growth, inadequate intake and social problems, are detected through the history (Weinzimmer & Schwartz, pp. 263-270).

19. **(d)** A common side effect of stimulants is a small increase in heart rate or blood pressure (Mercugliano, p. 872).

20. **(b)** Children with chronic medical illness typically strive actively to remain in school. The other findings listed in the other answer choices are more likely to be associated with school phobia (Hodas, 1997b, p. 941).

21. **(a)** Excessive eating followed by purging is a sign of bulimia (Sargent, 1997b, p. 935)

References

Curry, T. A. (1997). Problems of newborn care. In M. W. Schwartz, T. A. Curry, A. J. Sargent, N. J. Blum, & J. A. Fein (Eds.), *Pediatric primary care: A problem oriented approach* (3rd ed., pp. 43-54). St. Louis: Mosby.

Eiger, M. S. (1997). Feeding of infants and children. In R. A. Hoekelman, S. B. Friedman, N. M. Nelson, H. M. Seidel, & M. L. Weitzman (Eds.), *Primary pediatric care* (3rd ed., pp. 168-181). St. Louis: Mosby.

Grundy, J. H. (1997). The pediatric physical examination. In R. A. Hoekelman, S. B. Friedman, N. M. Nelson, H. M. Seidel, & M. L. Weitzman (Eds.), *Primary pediatric care* (3rd ed., pp. 55-98). St. Louis: Mosby.

Hodas, G. R. (1997a). Depression. In M. W. Schwartz, T. A. Curry, A. J. Sargent, N. J. Blum, & J. A. Fein (Eds.), *Pediatric primary care: A problem-oriented approach* (3rd ed., pp. 918-921). St. Louis: Mosby.

Hodas, G. R. (1997b). School refusal. In M. W. Schwartz, T. A. Curry, A. J. Sargent, N. J. Blum, & J. A. Fein (Eds.), *Pediatric primary care: A problem-oriented approach* (3rd ed., pp. 940-942). St. Louis: Mosby.

Holtzman, N. A., & Braverman, N. E. (1997). Recognition of genetic-metabolic diseases by clinical diagnosis and screening. In R. A. Hoekelman, S. B. Friedman, N. M. Nelson, H. M. Seidel, & M. L. Weitzman (Eds.), *Primary pediatric care* (3rd ed., pp. 204-216). St. Louis: Mosby.

Mercugliano, M. (1997). Attention deficit hyperactivity disorder. In M. W. Schwartz, T. A. Curry, A. J. Sargent, N. J. Blum, & J. A. Fein (Eds.), *Pediatric primary care: A problem-oriented approach* (3rd ed., pp. 868-873). St. Louis: Mosby.

Poncz, M. (1997). Anemia. In M. W. Schwartz, T. A. Curry, A. J. Sargent, N. J. Blum, & J.A. Fein (Eds.), *Pediatric primary care: A problem-oriented approach* (3rd ed., pp. 585-595). St. Louis: Mosby.

Sargent, J. (1997a). Drug and alcohol abuse. In M. W. Schwartz, T. A. Curry, A. J. Sargent, N. J. Blum, & J. A. Fein (Eds.), *Pediatric primary care: A problem-oriented approach* (3rd ed., pp. 926-932). St. Louis: Mosby.

Sargent, J. (1997b). Eating disorders. In M. W. Schwartz, T. A. Curry, A. J. Sargent, N. J. Blum, & J. A. Fein (Eds.), *Pediatric primary care: A problem-oriented approach* (3rd ed., pp. 933-939). St. Louis: Mosby.

Seidl, T. (1997). Child abuse and neglect. In M. W. Schwartz, T. A. Curry, A. J. Sargent, N. J. Blum, & J. A. Fein (Eds.), *Pediatric primary care: A problem-oriented approach* (3rd ed., pp. 976-979). St. Louis: Mosby.

Simeonsson, R. J., & Simeonsson, N. (1997). Developmental surveillance and intervention. In R. A. Hoekelman, S. B. Friedman, N. M. Nelson, H. M. Seidel, & M. L. Weitzman (Eds.), *Primary pediatric care* (3rd ed., pp. 236-243). St. Louis: Mosby.

Simoes, E. A., & Groothuis, J. R. (1997) Immunization. In W. W. Hay, Jr., J. R. Groothuis, A. R. Hayward, & M. J. Levin (Eds.), *Current pediatric diagnosis and treatment* (13th ed., pp. 234-259). Stamford, CT: Appleton & Lange.

Weinzimmer, S. A., & Schwartz, M. W. (1997). Growth problems. In M. W. Schwartz, T. A. Curry, A. J. Sargent, N. J. Blum, & J. A. Fein (Eds.), *Pediatric primary care: A problem-oriented approach* (3rd ed., pp. 263-270). St. Louis: Mosby.

Eye, Ear, Nose, and Throat Disorders

Brenda Holloway

Select one best answer to the following questions

1. Following an episode of meningitis, it is most important to assess the child for:
   - a. Hearing loss
   - b. Change in taste
   - c. Cervical lymphadenopathy
   - d. Tinnitus

2. An 8-year-old has been brought to the clinic with a chief complaint of ear pain. When you grasp the pinna of the ear, he says "that hurts real bad." These findings are consistent with a diagnosis of:
   - a. Serous otitis media
   - b. Mastoiditis
   - c. Otitis externa
   - d. Cholesteatoma

3. Ten-year-old Steven has been diagnosed with otitis externa twice this year. Health teaching for Steven and his mother should include:
   - a. Emphasis on consistent use of low dose prophylactic antibiotics
   - b. Sleeping with the affected ear in the dependent position
   - c. Information on the use of decongestants to open the eustachian tube
   - d. Information on the use of acetic acid after ear canal contact with water

4. Following tympanostomy tube insertion, it is important that the tubes remain patent. Which of the following methods may be used to determine patency?
   - a. Visual inspection
   - b. Impedance tympanometry

    c. Valsalva maneuver

    d. Instillation of an ototopical suspension

5. The diagnosis of acute otitis media in a 1-year-old is based on:

    a. Abnormal findings when pneumatic otoscopy and hearing test are performed

    — b. Changes in the tympanic membrane's contour, color, and mobility

    c. Presence of fever and color of the tympanic membrane

    d. Presence of fever, ear pain, and tenderness of the pinna

6. Twelve-month-old Connor has been treated five times for acute otitis media. When planning Conner's follow-up care, it is most important to evaluate for which of the following?

    a. Otitis externa

    — b. Hearing loss

    c. Enlarged tonsils

    d. Shotty lymph nodes

7. Thirteen-year-old Brian presents to the clinic with a sore throat. History reveals that he had a sore throat a couple of weeks ago and thought he had gotten well. He now has severe pharyngeal pain of two days duration and says he has been sweating and thinks he has fever. Physical examination reveals a temperature of 102° F and erythematous and edematous pharynx and soft palate. The right tonsil is swollen and inflamed without exudate and the uvula is displaced to the left. Right cervical nodes are tender. Lungs are clear to auscultation. Brian's signs and symptoms are suggestive of:

    a. Acute uvulitis

    b. Viral pharyngitis

    c. Epiglottitis

    — d. Peritonsillar abscess

8. Which of the following is an expected finding after treatment of acute suppurative otitis media?

    a. Otitis externa

    b. Central auditory dysfunction

    c. Functional hearing loss

    — d. Middle ear effusion

9. Two-year-old Shanda's mother has brought her to the clinic because she thinks

the child is having trouble hearing. Your evaluation of the complaint should start with:

— a. Asking detailed questions related to Shanda's medical history
  b. Examination of the ear
  c. Tympanometry and hearing tests
  d. Assuring Shanda's mother that transient hearing loss in childhood is common

10. Assessment of the red reflex may be used to rule out which of the following?

  a. Opacities
  b. Myopia or hyperopia
  c. Decreased visual acuity
  d. Blindness

11. The mother of 2-year-old Bridget has brought her to the clinic because "she got bathroom cleanser in her eye." History reveals that about 30 minutes ago Bridget was sitting on the floor playing with a squeeze bottle of bathroom cleaner, when the bottle accidently opened and the liquid splashed into her right eye. Physical examination reveals a reddened right eye with an edematous lid. Initial treatment should include:

  a. Reassuring the mother and allowing the natural tearing process to cleanse the eye
  b. Performing a retinal fundoscopic examination to assess for burns
— c. Irrigating the eye with copious amount of normal saline
  d. Having Bridget's mother take her to an ophthalmologist

12. The mother of a 5-year-old child has brought him to the clinic because she thinks he has "pink eye." Which of the following would lead you to consider a diagnosis other than bacterial conjunctivitis?

  a. Hyperemic conjunctiva
  b. Scratchy sensation in the eye
  c. Decreased corneal clarity
  d. Copious tearing

13. Eighteen-month-old Julie has been brought to the clinic by her mother who tells you that Julie has had a "cold" for the past four days. There is no history of cough and the mother is unsure whether Julie has had fever. Physical examination reveals greenish, blood-tinged mucus with a strong, foul odor, draining

from the right nostril. This clinical picture is most consistent with a diagnosis of:

    a. Allergic rhinitis
    b. Viral rhinitis
    c. Acute sinusitis
  — d. Nasal foreign body

14. In a child with chronic sinusitis, the most accurate method of identifying sinus abnormalities is:

    a. Dark room transillumination of the sinuses *no*
    b. Percussion of the paranasal sinuses *no*
    c. AP, lateral, and occipitomental sinus radiographs *no*
    d. CT scan of the sinuses

Questions 15 and 16 refer to the following scenario.

Ten-year-old Mike has been brought to the clinic with "a cold." History reveals that he has had a runny nose and cough for about 10 days. There is no history of frequent respiratory problems. Physical examination reveals a temperature of 100° F and edematous cervical lymph nodes. Eyes are without redness or swelling. Examination of the nose is significant for mucopurulent drainage from the middle meatus bilaterally. The pharynx is erythematous without tonsillar enlargement or exudate. Breath is malodorous and lungs are clear to auscultation.

15. Mike's management should include:

    a. Culture of the nasal drainage
    b. Radiograph of the sinuses
    c. Measurement of erythrocyte sedimentation rate
  — d. Use of an antibiotic

16. Two days after Mike's first visit, his mother brings him back to the clinic because he has a "swollen eye." Observation reveals redness and inflammation of the right eyelid with impaired extraocular movement. Which action is appropriate?

    a. Reassure the mother that this is a common and usually benign condition
    b. Treat Mike for bacterial conjunctivitis
    c. Order anti-inflammatory eye drops
  — d. Refer Mike immediately to a pediatrician

17. Twelve-year-old Nathan's mother has brought him to the clinic because he has had a runny nose for two weeks. History reveals that Nathan has visited the clinic three other times this year for upper respiratory complaints. Examination reveals slightly edematous and erythematous eyes, pale nasal mucosa with clear mucus, and pharynx with thin secretions posteriorly. There is no tonsillar swelling or exudate. Lips and nail beds are pink. Lymph node examination is significant for multiple shotty nodes. Lungs are clear to auscultation. Which action is appropriate at this time?

    a. Discuss symptomatic relief of the common cold with Nathan and his mother
    b. Culture nasal drainage and delay treatment until results are known
    c. Order an antibiotic
    d. Order an antihistamine   *allergies*

18. A 1-week-old infant has been diagnosed with nasolacrimal duct obstruction. Usual initial therapy includes:

    a. Use of prophylactic antibiotics
    b. Nasolacrimal sac massage
    c. Surgical opening of obstructed ducts
    d. Referral to an ophthalmologist

19. Four-year-old Marie has been brought to the clinic because she "has something wrong with her eye." Marie and her mother report that there has been no injury to the eye and that it has been red since yesterday. Examination reveals conjunctival hyperemia and a copious amount of purulent discharge bilaterally. Vision, pupillary reflexes, and corneal clarity are all normal. Which treatment should be ordered?

    a. Sodium sulfacetamide ophthalmic solution *- bacterial conjunctivitis*
    b. Gentamycin ophthalmic solution *gram ⊖ bacteria or Cx results*
    c. Tobramycin ophthalmic solution
    d. Cromolyn sodium ophthalmic solution *- allergic conjunctivitis*

20. During the routine examination of a 12-year-old boy, you detect a group of hard, fixed, non-tender lymph nodes, each of which measure about one centimeter, in the posterior cervical chain. You are unable to detect any signs of infection. Your management should include:

    a. Recording the finding and reassessing the nodes in one month
    b. Ordering a 10 day course of a broad spectrum antibiotic and re-evaluating the nodes in two weeks

— c. Ordering a CBC, erythrocyte sedimentation rate, and chest radiograph
d. Referring the child to an allergist

21. Which method might be used to assess the vision of a 1-month-old?

    a. Check the vessel pattern of the fundus of the eye
    b. Watch to see if the infant turns his head toward you when you speak
    c. Observe the pattern of interaction with the mother
    d. Perform the Titmus test on the infant

Answers and Rationale

1. **(a)** Complications of meningitis include hydrocephalus, deafness, and blindness (Hoekelman, et al., p. 992).

2. **(c)** With otitis externa, exquisite tenderness is noted when pressure is placed on the tragus or pinna of the ear (Hoekelman, et al., p. 1475).

3. **(d)** Otitis externa may be prevented by instilling 2% acetic acid (half strength vinegar) in the external auditory canal after ear canal contact with water (Hoekelman, et al., p. 1475).

4. **(a)** Visual inspection is used to determine tube patency (Hoekelman, et al., p. 1475).

5. **(b)** The diagnosis of acute otitis media is based on changes in the contour, color, and mobility of the tympanic membrane. Redness of the tympanic membrane alone can be caused by crying and is not a reliable sign of acute otitis media. Changes in contour, mobility, and hearing may be caused by nonsuppurative or serous otitis media. Fever, ear pain, and tenderness of the pinna may indicate otitis externa (Hoekelman, et al., p. 1473).

6. **(b)** Hearing loss is the most common complication of otitis media. Children who have multiple infections should have their hearing assessed. Tonsils are normally large in young children. Shotty lymph nodes are usually associated with past infections and are not clinically significant (Hoekelman, et al., p. 1475).

7. **(d)** This presentation is classical for peritonsillar abscess which is generally treated with incision and drainage and antibiotics (Behrman, et al., p. 1192; Oski, et al., pp. 970-971)

8. **(d)** Middle ear effusion (serous otitis media) is frequently seen after acute otitis media. Central auditory dysfunction is caused by the brain's inability to use sound properly. Functional hearing loss means there is no disturbance with any organ and may be psychiatric in origin (Hoekelman, et al., pp. 992, 1274).

9. **(a)** The investigation of all complaints begins with exploration of the history. Hearing loss in childhood is extremely common. Specific historical risk factors for hearing loss are family history of congenital hearing loss, prenatal or perinatal infection, birth trauma or anoxia, and use of aminoglycosides (Hoekelman, et al., p. 991).

10. **(a)** A normal red reflex rules out opacities, intraocular tumor, and coloboma. The red reflex does not assess visual acuity. A non-visible red reflex indicates obstruction in the preretinal chambers (Oski, et al., pp. 44, 1148).

11. **(c)** Acid or alkali chemical eye injuries are acute emergencies and require copious normal saline. Over irrigation is not a problem but litmus paper can be used to determine when the chemical has been neutralized. The child should be referred to an ophthalmologist after irrigation of the eye (Oski, et al., p. 887; Hoekelman, et al., p. 1462).

12. **(c)** Bacterial conjunctivitis does not affect corneal clarity. A more serious condition should be suspected (such as keratitis, corneal ulcer, or glaucoma) and the child referred to an ophthalmologist if the cornea is not clear (Oski, et al., p. 886-887; Hoekelman, et al., p. 1095).

13. **(d)** Nasal foreign body is characterized by unilateral purulent discharge that may be blood tinged. Nasal discharge is very foul smelling. Allergic rhinitis and viral rhinitis usually cause clear bilateral nasal secretions, while sinusitis usually produces bilateral drainage with less odor (Oski, et al., p. 953)

14. **(d)** CT scans are superior to sinus radiographs in the identification of abnormalities. A normal radiograph suggests, but does not prove, that sinuses are disease free (Oski, et al., p. 953).

15. **(d)** The signs and symptoms, especially mucopurulent drainage from the middle meatus, are supportive of a diagnosis of acute sinusitis. Sinus radiographs are difficult to interpret and not indicated at this time. Culture of nasal drainage is not useful in the determination of the causative organism in sinusitis. There are no signs of complications, and it is appropriate to treat the condition with antibiotics (Behrman, et al., p. 1192-1193; Oski, et al., p. 953).

16. **(d)** History of sinusitis often precedes orbital cellulitis. Examination indicates that Mike may have orbital cellulitis which is a medical emergency that requires hospitalization and IV antibiotics. He should be referred to a physician for evaluation (Hoekelman, et al., pp. 1535-1536; Oski, et al., p. 887).

17. **(d)** Repeated episodes of upper respiratory illness, clear nasal secretions, and pale nasal mucosa are common in children with allergies. Antihistamines are used to treat seasonal and perennial allergies (Behrman, et al., p. 626-627).

18. **(b)** Nasolacrimal sac massage using downward strokes raises the pressure in the nasolacrimal sac and may overcome the obstruction. Prophylactic or long term antibiotics are not advised. Early surgical opening of the ducts may be performed to relieve parental anxiety but conservative treatment is successful by one year of age in about 90% of cases. Referral to an ophthalmologist is indicated if the condition persists beyond six months or is frequently purulent (Hoekelman, et al., pp. 1097-1098).

19. **(a)** Marie's presentation supports a diagnosis of bacterial conjunctivitis. Sodium sulfacetamide, erythromycin, or polymixin B sulfate-trimethoprim sulfate solution are appropriate first line treatments. Gentamycin and tobramycin should be reserved for suspected gram negative bacterial conjunctivitis or when justified by culture results. Cromolyn sodium is used to treat allergic conjunctivitis (Hoekelman, et al., pp. 1094-1095; Oski, et al., p. 886).

20. **(c)** Nodes that are matted, hard, fixed, and non-tender are characteristic of cancer. Lymph nodes associated with Hodgkin's disease usually begin in the lower cervical area. A chest radiograph, CBC, and erythrocyte sedimentation rate should be obtained in any patient with lymphadenopathy that is atypical for infection (Thompson & Wilson, p. 172; Hoekelman, et al., pp. 1231-1232).

21. **(c)** Nonquantitative but clinically helpful information may be gained about the infant's vision by observing whether the infant fixates on and attempts to follow the mother's face (Oski, et al., p. 878).

References

Behrman, R. E., Kliegman, R. M., & Arvin, A. M. (1996). *Nelson textbook of pediatrics* (15th ed.). Philadelphia: W. B. Saunders.

Hoekelman, R. A., Friedman, S. B., Nelson, N. M., Seidel, H. M., & Weitzman, M. L. (Eds.). (1997). *Primary pediatric care* (3rd ed.). St. Louis: Mosby.

Oski, L. A., DeAngelis, C. D., Feigin, R. D., McMillan, J. A., & Warshaw, J. B. (Eds.). (1994). *Principles and practice of pediatrics.* Philadelphia: J. B. Lippincott.

Thompson, J. M., & Wilson, S. F. (1996). *Health assessment for nursing practice.* St. Louis: Mosby.

Cardiovascular Disorders

Brenda Holloway

Select one best answer to the following questions.

1. In the infant, child, or adolescent, which of the following is considered by the Second Task Force on Blood Pressure Control in Children to be diagnostic for high blood pressure? Three blood pressure readings above the:

   a. 50th percentile for height and weight
   b. 75th percentile for weight and sex
   c. 80th percentile for age and race
   d. 95th percentile for age and sex

2. Based on knowledge of the most common causes of hypertension in young children, initial diagnostic laboratory evaluation for a 4-year-old with high blood pressure must include which of the following?

   a. Blood glucose measurement
   b. Echocardiogram
   c. Liver enzymes
   d. Urinalysis

3. A child's arm is five inches in length from the elbow to the olecranon process, and average in circumference. Which of the following available blood pressure cuffs should be used to assess the child's blood pressure?

   a. A one inch cuff
   b. A two inch cuff
   c. A three inch cuff
   d. A four inch cuff   *should cover 75% of upper arm*

4. When assessing blood pressure in a 4-year-old child, you note that the diastolic sound becomes muffled at 40 mm Hg but is audible to 0 mm Hg. Which of the following is true?

a. 0 mm Hg should be considered the diastolic pressure
b. 40 mm Hg should be considered the diastolic pressure
c. A diastolic reading is usually not assessed in children
d. The child should be referred to a cardiologist

Questions 5 and 6 refer to the following scenario.

5. The mother of 4-day-old Ethan has brought him to the clinic because he is not eating well. The infant's hospital record indicates that he was born at 40 weeks gestation and although all vital signs were normal and his color was pink, a grade III/VI cardiac murmur was noted at discharge. You observe that the infant's lips and nail beds are now bluish and his respiratory rate is 90 breaths per minute. A grade IV/VI holosystolic murmur is heard best along the lower left sternal border. Differential diagnosis should include:

a. Respiratory distress syndrome
b. A right-to-left cardiac shunt *cyanotic*
c. Mitral regurgitation
d. Patent ductus arteriosus *acyanotic*

6. Laboratory studies are ordered for baby Ethan. Which finding should be considered <u>abnormal</u>?

a. A chest radiograph that reveals that the heart occupies 50% of the cardiothoracic dimension *nl*
b. A chest radiograph that reveals vascular markings in the peripheral $\frac{1}{3}$ of the lung fields *nl*
c. An ECG reveals a sustained resting heart rate of 190 beats per minute
d. An ECG indicates right ventricular dominance *nl*

7. The mother of a 4-week-old infant has brought him to the clinic because he is eating poorly and looks "puffy." Examination reveals a lethargic infant with generalized edema. Based on knowledge of the most common causes of generalized edema in infancy, an appropriate initial diagnostic test would be a(n):

a. Chest radiograph *to confirm CHF – edema*
b. ASO titre
c. Sickle cell prep
d. RBC with indices

8. During the routine physical examination of a 3-year-old child, cardiac auscultation reveals an irregular heartbeat of 90 beats per minute that slows when the

respiratory rate slows and accelerates when the child breathes faster. Physical examination findings are otherwise negative. Which of the following is an appropriate response to his finding?

- a. Record the findings in the child's record
- b. Order a chest radiograph
- c. Order an echocardiogram
- d. Refer the child to a cardiologist

9. A child with Wolff-Parkinson-White syndrome is being treated with propranolol. Effectiveness of treatment is determined by evaluating which of the following?

- a. Blood pressure
- b. Cyanotic episodes
- c. Activity level
- d. Heart rate

10. A 7-year-old child presents to the clinic for his initial visit with a chief complaint of earache. Medical history is negative except for numerous episodes of "ear infections." Physical findings include an oral temperature of 103° F, a red and bulging right tympanic membrane, and a grade III/VI systolic cardiac murmur. The child is at approximately the 50th percentile for weight and the 60th percentile for height. In addition to recording the finding, what action should the PNP take regarding the murmur?

- a. Order an ECG
- b. Order an echocardiogram
- c. Order an RBC with indices
- d. Re-evaluate the murmur in two weeks   *when afebrile*

11. While examining a 3-month-old girl, you note a grade III/VI ejection heart murmur that is heard best at the second intercostal space, left sternal border. This finding should be further investigated to rule out:

- a. Tetralogy of Fallot   *pulmonary stenosis*
- b. Patent ductus arteriosus
- c. Mitral valve prolapse
- d. Wolff-Parkinson-White syndrome

12. A 4-year-old boy has presented to the clinic with signs and symptoms of Kawasaki disease. Initial management should include:

- a. Teaching the mother to monitor for complications at home

b. Supportive home therapy with a high protein diet
c. Isolation and identification of pre-school aged contacts
d. Hospitalization and bed rest

13. Which of the following drugs is important in the management of symptoms, and the prevention of complications from, Kawasaki disease?

a. Aspirin
b. Corticosteroids
c. Acetaminophen
d. Penicillin

14. An 8-year-old female has just been diagnosed with rheumatic fever. Initial management should include initiation of:

a. An anti-inflammatory agent and activity as tolerated
b. Penicillin and return to school within 48 hours
c. Penicillin and isolation from contact with other children until afebrile
d. An anti-inflammatory agent and bed rest

15. In the management of rheumatic fever, which laboratory test may be used to validate decreasing inflammation?

a. Antistreptolysin O titre
b. Throat culture
c. Erythrocyte sedimentation rate
d. The Duckett Jones test

Answers and Rationale

1. **(d)** High blood pressure is defined by the Second Task Force on Blood Pressure Control in Children as three blood pressure readings above the 95th percentile for age and sex (Hoekelman, et al., p. 217).

2. **(d)** Initial diagnostic laboratory work for the young child with hypertension is based on the fact that renal problems are a predominant cause of hypertension in this age group (Hoekelman, et al., p. 217).

3. **(d)** The blood pressure cuff width should cover approximately 75% of the upper arm (Hoekelman, et al., p. 217).

4. **(b)** The muffling phase (K4) should be used as the diastolic blood pressure in young children because disappearance of sound (K5) may not occur in this age group (Hoekelman, et al., p. 217).

5. **(b)** Symptoms of a right to left shunt (except for a murmur) are often not noticeable until several days after birth when the ductus arteriosus closes. Cyanosis is secondary to decreased pulmonary blood flow as the deoxygenated blood on the right side of the heart shunts to the left side of the heart and then enters the peripheral circulation. Respiratory distress syndrome is noted within hours after birth. Patent ductus arteriosus is an acyanotic heart condition. Mitral regurgitation is not a cyanotic heart condition (Hoekelman, et al., p. 1253).

6. **(c)** A sustained resting heart rate above 180 bpm is above normal limits. Answers "a," "b," and "d" indicate normal findings for this age group (Hoekelman, et al., pp. 531, 1253).

7. **(a)** Congenital heart disease is a common cause of edema in infancy. Heart failure can be confirmed with chest radiograph. If poststreptococcal glomerulonephritis were suspected, an ASO titre would be ordered. This condition is rare in infancy. Sickle cell disease rarely causes problems in infancy (Hoekelman, et al., pp. 933-934).

8. **(a)** Normal sinus arrhythmia is the most common cause of an irregular heartbeat in children and is characterized by a rate that slows and accelerates in

response to changes in respiratory rate. This is a normal finding (Hoekel-man, et al., p. 115).

9. **(d)** Wolff-Parkinson-White is a cause of supraventricular tachycardia. Proprano-lol may be used to slow the heart rate (Hoekelman, et al., p. 881).

10. **(d)** Murmurs are the result of turbulent blood flow. Turbulence may be caused by conditions which increase blood flow to the heart, such as fever. Since the child's growth is within normal limits and there appear to be no other negative cardiac findings, the murmur should be re-evaluated when the child is afebrile (Jarvis, p. 543).

11. **(a)** Advancing Tetralogy of Fallot results in right ventricular outflow obstruc-tion (pulmonary stenosis). An ejection murmur indicates turbulence as blood flows through a narrowed orifice or semilunar valve as blood leaves the heart. The aortic and pulmonic valves are the semilunar valves. Other answers do not involve semilunar valves (Hoekelman, et al., pp. 994, 1254).

12. **(d)** Children with Kawasaki disease are usually hospitalized due to irritability, fever, and the need for IV fluids. Bed rest is recommended until the 2nd or 3rd week after the onset of fever because of myocarditis associated with the disease (Oski, et al., p. 1426).

13. **(a)** Aspirin helps reduce the fever associated with Kawasaki disease, and has been shown to reduce the rate of aneurysm development. Most deaths from Kawasaki disease are attributed to coronary artery thrombosis (Oski, et al., pp. 1425-1426).

14. **(d)** Anti-inflammatory agents are used in the treatment of rheumatic fever. An antibiotic (often penicillin) is given, but bedrest is recommended until in-flammation subsides (Oski, et al., p. 1631).

15. **(c)** A declining erythrocyte sedimentation rate (ESR or sedimentation rate) indi-cates decreasing inflammatory activity which indicates that increased physi-cal activity may be tolerated (Hoekelman, et al., p. 1551).

References

Hoekelman, R. A., Friedman, S. B., Nelson, N. M., Seidel, H. M., & Weitzman, M. L. (Eds.). (1997). *Primary pediatric care* (3rd ed.). St. Louis: Mosby.

Jarvis, C. (1996). *Physical examination and health assessment.* Philadelphia: W. B. Saunders.

Oski, F. A., DeAngelis, C. D., Feigin, R. D., McMillan, J. A., & Warshaw, J. B. (Eds.). (1994). *Principles and practice of pediatrics.* Philadelphia: J. B. Lippincott.

Respiratory Disorders

Brenda Holloway

Select one best answer to the following questions.

1. The PNP is teaching a group of expectant parents about infant care and illness prevention. It is most important for the PNP to stress:

    a. Keeping all animals out of the house
    b. Keeping the infant away from cigarette smoke
    c. Keeping the infant well covered at night
    d. Keeping the infant away from crowds

2. Which of the following does not place the infant at increased risk for sudden infant death syndrome?

    a. Documented episodes of periodic breathing — nl in infants
    b. Prematurity
    c. Severe bronchopulmonary dysplasia
    d. Apnea of prematurity

3. In the management of a child with bronchiolitis, the early use of which of the following is likely to be the most beneficial?

    a. Antihistamines
    b. Broad spectrum antibiotics
    c. Sedating type cough suppressants
    d. Bronchodilators

4. A NICU graduate with bronchopulmonary dysplasia (BPD) has been discharged to home. A potential problem area that requires close monitoring is:

    a. Insufficient caloric intake
    b. Atrophy of abdominal muscles due to abdominal breathing patterns
    c. Lack of tactile stimuli due to restrictions on parental handling
    d. The predisposition to development of nasal polyps

5. A 10-day-old infant has been brought to the clinic by his mother because his nose has been running and he has had a dry cough without fever for the past two days. The mother tells you that she had two cousins who died with cystic fibrosis, and that she wants a sweat test performed on her baby. Your <u>initial response should be to examine the baby and</u>:

    a. Assure the mother that the baby is too young to be suffering from cystic fibrosis

    b. Assure the mother that cystic fibrosis is not inherited

    c. Schedule testing to be done when the baby is older

    d. Refer the baby to a pulmonologist for thorough evaluation

6. To promote normal growth in the child with cystic fibrosis, dietary management should include:

    a. Limited fats and 50% more calories than usual daily allowances

    b. Liberal fats and 50% more calories than usual daily allowances

    c. The usual number of calories as indicated by height and weight plus fat soluble vitamins

    d. Limited fat and sodium in moderation

7. Mrs. S. has brought 10-day-old Jacob to the clinic because she is concerned about his breathing. She says that while she is feeding the baby, he often stops breathing for periods of about 10 seconds. History reveals that Jacob eats well, has never appeared pale or cyanotic, and has never become limp during any of the apnea episodes. Your management plan is based on the knowledge that:

    a. This is a normal breathing pattern for an infant

    b. These episodes likely indicate aspiration of formula and should be evaluated

    c. A variety of pathological processes are associated with the episodes described

    d. Neurological deficits in infants are often manifested by such episodes

Questions 8 and 9 refer to the following scenario.

Four-year-old Julie has a history of asthma. Her mother brings her to the clinic and states that Julie has been coughing and wheezing severely for the past 10 hours. Physical examination reveals a respiratory rate of 14 breaths per minute. Respirations are shallow without wheezing and there are no retractions.

8. What is the most likely reason that wheezing is not auscultated?

    a. Julie is upset about something and has faked an asthma attack
    b. Julie's mother needs education regarding identification of wheezing
    c. Julie's condition has improved significantly
    d. Wheezes are not being generated because breathing is shallow
       nl resp rate for a 4 y.o. is 20-30 bpm

9. Appropriate initial management of Julie's condition is to:

    a. Talk with Julie alone and ask what is upsetting her
    b. Educate the mother regarding identification of wheezing
    c. Tell Julie's mother to continue with treatment that has been effective in the past
    d. Administer a bronchodilator

10. Five-month-old Matthew is brought to the clinic because he has been coughing and has had clear rhinorrhea for the last two days. His mother tells you that he has never been sick before. Family history is positive for allergies and you hear generalized wheezing. You may conclude that:

    a. Matthew has familial asthma
    b. Matthew has asthma exacerbated by a viral infection
    c. Matthew should be referred for allergy testing
    d. Asthma should not be diagnosed at this stage

11. When educating parents regarding transmission of respiratory syncytial virus (RSV), it is important to stress that:

    a. Children with RSV should be totally isolated from other children
    b. RSV is usually spread by airborne particles
    c. Children who attend day care centers should take prophylactic antibiotics early each fall
    d. Hand washing is the most effective procedure in the prevention of RSV transmission

12. In mild to moderate attacks of acute asthma, albuterol should be given every 3 to 4 hours and routine medications should be:

    a. Continued as usual
    b. Discontinued until albuterol treatments are deemed unnecessary
    c. Given only if the albuterol is ineffective
    d. Be decreased to the minimum recommended dose

Questions 13 and 14 refer to the following scenario.

Seven-year-old Josh presents to the clinic with inspiratory stridor, drooling, and a temperature of 105° F. He insists on sitting up during the clinical examination.

13. This clinical picture is most consistent with a diagnosis of:

    a. Aspirated foreign body no
    b. Reactive airway disease no
    c. Viral croup no
    d. Epiglottitis

14. Appropriate initial management of Josh includes:

    a. High doses of an oral broad spectrum antibiotic and antipyretics no
    b. Teaching the mother to administer racemic epinephrine by nebulization no
    c. Teaching the mother how to administer loading and decreasing doses of prednisone no
    d. Immediate hospitalization with intravenous antibiotics

15. A diagnosis of croup is substantiated by which radiographic finding?

    a. Ground glass appearance in the upper airway
    b. Sparse areas of atelectasis
    c. "Thumb sign" on lateral view
    d. "Hourglass" narrowing in the subglottic region (steeple sign)

16. A lethargic appearing 18-month-old presents to the clinic with signs and symptoms of croup. Physical examination reveals a respiratory rate of 20 bpm and mild dehydration. Appropriate management includes: fatigue

    a. Instructing the mother to force fluids and use a cool mist humidifier in the child's room
    b. Instructing the mother to give fluids ad. lib. and to encourage intake of solid food
    c. Prescribing an oral broad spectrum antibiotic and prednisone
    d. Referring the child for hospitalization and IV fluids

17. A six-month-old boy is brought to the clinic because he has been coughing since yesterday. His mother states that he has never been sick before. She thinks he has been febrile but isn't sure. Physical examination reveals a well developed baby with a respiratory rate of 50 bpm, mild retractions, wheezes, and a dry cough. Chest radiograph reveals diffuse hyperinflation and patchy areas of infiltration. These findings are most consistent with a diagnosis of:

a. Laryngotracheobronchitis
b. Cystic fibrosis
c. Bronchiolitis
d. Respiratory distress syndrome

Questions 18 and 19 refer to the following scenario.

Twenty-two-month old Brent has been brought to the clinic by his mother who says he has been coughing for two days, and is now making a funny noise when he breathes. Examination reveals a fussy child with a brassy cough and inspiratory stridor. Lips and nail beds are pink. Axillary temperature is 103° F and respiratory rate is 50 bpm.

18. The most likely diagnosis of Brent's condition is:

    a. Laryngotracheobronchitis
    b. Bronchiolitis lung
    c. Respiratory distress syndrome lung
    d. Reactive airway disease lung

19. Which diagnostic test should be ordered first for Brent?

    a. Pulmonary function tests
    b. Throat culture
    c. Radiograph of the upper airway
    d. Laryngoscopic examination

20. Four-year-old Emily stays with her great aunt during the day while her mother is at work. Emily's mother has brought her to the clinic because the great aunt has just been diagnosed with TB. Emily's Mantoux skin test is positive but there is no clinical or radiographic evidence of disease. Appropriate management includes:

    a. Reassuring Emily's mother that no treatment is needed
    b. Administering another skin test in three months
    c. Oral penicillin therapy
    d. Oral preventive isoniazid therapy

Questions 21, 22, and 23 refer to the following scenario.

Two-year-old Heather's mother has brought her to the clinic with a "bad cough." History reveals onset of illness four days ago with clear rhinorrhea and coughing.

Her mother says that Heather's fever has been as high as 103° F under the arm. Physical examination reveals a temperature of 101° F (axillary) and respiratory rate of 56 bpm, with slight nasal flaring and intercostal, subcostal, and suprasternal retractions. The pharynx is red without tonsillar exudate. Chest auscultation reveals widespread rales and wheezing. The lips and nail beds are slightly pale but pink, skin turgor is good, and mucous membranes are moist.

21. The most likely diagnosis of Heather's condition is:

    a. Viral pneumonia
    b. Pneumococcal pneumonia
    c. Streptococcal pneumonia
    d. *Haemophilus influenzeae* type b pneumonia

22. Initially Heather should receive which diagnostic test?

    a. Sputum culture
    b. Sputum gram stain
    c. Chest radiograph
    d. Erythrocyte sedimentation rate

23. When deciding whether Heather should be treated at home or in the hospital, it is most important to consider Heather's:

    a. Maximum temperature
    b. Frequency of coughing episodes
    c. Hydration status
    d. Total length of illness

Answers and Rationale

1. **(b)** Exposure to cigarette smoke has been associated with increased incidence of illnesses such as asthma, bronchiolitis, and otitis media in children. None of the other options is as strongly associated with childhood illness (Behrman, et al., pp. 619, 1210-1212, 1815, 1994).

2. **(a)** Infantile apnea or periodic breathing (periods of less than 15 to 20 seconds) without pallor, cyanosis, or limpness is normal and is not related to SIDS. Other answers have been associated with increased incidence of SIDS (Hoekelman, et al., pp. 79, 538, 576-577).

3. **(d)** Many children with bronchiolitis benefit from the use of bronchodilators. Other medications listed have not been shown to be effective treatment (Hoekelman, et al., p. 827).

4. **(a)** The pathophysiology of BPD is similar to chronic obstructive lung disease (COLD). Diuretic use and limitation of fluids is often part of the management plan. Limitation of fluids may make it difficult to provide adequate caloric intake (Hoekelman, et al., p. 576).

5. **(c)** In the presence of suggestive symptoms, a sweat chloride level above 60 mEq/L is diagnostic for the inherited disease, cystic fibrosis. A sweat test performed in the first few weeks of life may be unreliable because of low sweat rates. An infant without obvious signs of serious illness should not be referred to a pulmonologist at age 10 days (Hoekelman, et al., p. 418).

6. **(b)** Because of steatorrhea and metabolic demands, the child with cystic fibrosis should receive 50% more calories than the usual daily allowance. Liberal fat should be allowed in the diet and may even be supplemented with MCT oil and polycose (Oski, et al., p. 1499).

7. **(a)** Brief apnea episodes (less than 15 to 20 seconds) are normal in infants and are most frequent in preterm infants. These normal episodes are not associated with pallor, cyanosis, or hypotonia (Hoekelman, et al., pp. 79, 533, 538, 576).

8. **(d)** A respiratory rate of 14 breaths per minute is slow for a four-year-old and

is an indicator that there is muscle fatigue or that the child is in extreme respiratory distress. When the wheezing child develops muscle fatigue, a wheeze may not be generated, even in the presence of severe obstruction (Behrman, et al., p. 630; Hoekelman, et al., p. 1159).

9. **(d)** When there are signs of muscle fatigue, and breathing is shallow in a known asthmatic, a bronchodilator should be given to help relieve airway obstruction (Behrman, et al., p. 630).

10. **(d)** Asthma is not diagnosed during a child's first episode of wheezing, but after a documented pattern of recurrent wheezing responsive to bronchodilator therapy. Differential diagnoses should include foreign body, congenital malformation, and bronchiolitis (Hoekelman, et al., pp. 1159-1160; Oski, et al., p. 827).

11. **(d)** Hand to nose or conjunctival mucosa, after touching an RSV contaminated fomite, is the chief means of RSV transmission (Oski, et al., p. 1300).

12. **(a)** Routine asthma medications should continue even when albuterol is needed (Oski, et al., p. 221).

13. **(d)** Epiglottitis usually occurs in children age 6 to 10 years, while croup usually occurs in children ages 3 months to 3 years. The child with epiglottitis runs a high fever, drools, and insists on sitting up, usually leaning forward in the "tripod" position (Hoekelman, et al., pp. 1702-1703).

14. **(d)** Epiglottitis progresses quickly and is a medical emergency. Initial therapy is hospitalization (Hoekelman, et al., pp. 1704-1705).

15. **(d)** Inflammation in the subglottic region causes narrowing resulting in an "hourglass" or "steeple" sign seen best on posteroanterior view (Hoekelman, et al., pp. 1664, 1707).

16. **(d)** A respiratory rate of 20 bpm in an 18-month-old, accompanied by lethargy and mild dehydration, likely indicates that the child has become fatigued from the increased effort of breathing. The child should be hospitalized

and given IV fluids to allow for rest and rehydration while respiratory status is closely monitored (Hoekelman, et al., p. 1665).

17. **(c)** The infant with bronchiolitis typically presents with low grade fever, cough, dyspnea, and wheezing. Chest radiograph reveals hyperinflation and perhaps patchy infiltrates. Laryngotracheobronchitis produces a barking cough without the stated radiograph findings. History of frequent illness is common with cystic fibrosis. Respiratory distress syndrome is a disease of the newborn (Oski, et al., pp. 1457-1458).

18. **(a)** Laryngotracheobronchitis (croup) is the most common cause of stridor. Stridor is usually caused by an upper airway condition. Other answers are not upper airway conditions (Behrman, et al., p. 1201.).

19. **(c)** Since stridor is usually caused by an upper airway condition, such as croup, epiglottitis, or foreign body aspiration, radiograph of the upper airway is helpful in diagnosing the cause of stridor. The invasive procedure, laryngoscopic examination, is dangerous and would not be used for initial diagnostic purposes (Behrman, et al., p. 1201; Burns, et al., p. 647).

20. **(d)** Isoniazid therapy is indicated if a child has a positive TB skin test and known exposure to TB even if there is no clinical or radiographic evidence of disease (AAP, p. 551).

21. **(a)** Respiratory viruses (particularly RSV, adenoviruses, parainfluenza virus types 1, 2, and 3), and enterovirus are the most common cause of pneumonia during the first several years of life. The condition is usually preceded by rhinitis and cough for several days. Temperatures with viral pneumonia are generally lower than with bacterial pneumonia. Rales and wheezing are common (Behrman, et al., p. 716; Burns, et al., p. 655).

22. **(c)** Pneumonia is diagnosed by chest radiograph. Other tests listed can indicate infection or inflammation, but not pneumonia specifically (Behrman, et al., p. 717; Burns, et al., p. 655).

23. **(c)** Children with viral pneumonia are usually treated at home with supportive measures unless they need intravenous fluids, oxygen or assisted ventilation (Behrman, et al., p. 717; Burns, et al., p. 655).

References

American Academy of Pediatrics (AAP). (1997). *Redbook: Report of the committee an infectious diseases* (24th ed.). Elk Grove Village, IL: Author.

Behrman, R. E., Kliegman, R. M., & Arvin, A. M. (Eds.). (1996). *Nelson textbook of pediatrics* (15th ed.). Philadelphia: W. B. Saunders.

Burns, C. E., Barber, N., Brady, M. A., & Dunn, A. M. (1996). *Pediatric primary care: A handbook for nurse practitioners.* Philadelphia: W. B. Saunders.

Hoekelman, R. A., Friedman, S. B., Nelson, N. M., Seidel, H. M., & Weitzman, M. L. (Eds.). (1997). *Primary pediatric care* (3rd ed.). St. Louis: Mosby.

Oski, F. A., DeAngelis, D. D., Feigin, R. D., McMillan, J. A., & Warshaw, J. B. (Eds.). (1994). *Principles and practice of pediatrics.* Philadelphia: J. B. Lippincott.

Dermatologic Disorders

Patricia Clinton

Select one best answer to the following questions.

1. A 7-year-old African-American female presents with several dry, raised, periungual lesions on the two middle fingers of her left hand. She has a history of nail biting. The most likely diagnosis is:

    a. Impetigo
    b. Molluscum contagiosum
    c. Common wart
    d. Herpetic whitlow

2. Which of the following secondary skin changes is not associated with atopic dermatitis?

    a. Lichenification
    b. Striae
    c. Hyperpigmentation
    d Crusting

3. In infants, the lesions associated with atopic dermatitis are most likely to appear on the:

    a. Cheeks and forehead   *infants*
    b. Wrists and ankles
    c. Antecubital and popliteal fossae
    d. Flexural surfaces   *children*

4. During your newborn examination of K.L. you note a generalized lacy reticulated blue discoloration. This clinical presentation describes:

    a. Harlequin color change
    b. Mongolian spots
    c. Blue nevus

(d.) Cutis marmorata

5. During 3-year-old J.T.'s physical examination you observe eight, light brown macules, ranging in size from 0.5 cm to 0.75 cm on his trunk, arms, and legs. Your management plan would be to:

   a. Educate the family to apply sunscreen frequently
   b. Explain that the lesions will fade with time
   (c.) Refer to a pediatrician
   d. Document the findings and re-evaluate in six months

6. Mrs. Franklin is concerned about a light pink lesion on the back of 2-month-old Aaron's neck that darkens with crying. This description is consistent with:

   a. Sturge-Weber disease
   (b.) Salmon patch
   c. Port-wine stain
   d. Strawberry mark

7. 7-year-old D.M. presents with a beefy red macular-papular rash in the diaper area with satellite lesions on the abdomen. The appropriate treatment would be:

   (a.) Clotrimazole   *candida albicans*
   b. A & D ointment
   c. Gentian violet 1% to 2%
   d. Hydrocortisone cream

Questions 8 and 9 refer to the following scenario.

4-month-old T.W.'s mother states that the infant has been irritable and not sleeping well. During the physical examination you note papular lesions on his feet and erythematous papules over his back.

8. To confirm your suspicion of scabies you would order a:

   a. Wood's lamp examination
   (b.) Microscopic skin scraping
   c. KOH preparation of skin scraping
   d. Skin culture

9. Having confirmed the diagnosis of scabies in T.W. the treatment of choice would be:

   (a.) Permethrin 5%

b. Lindane 1% *contraindicated*
c. Sulfur ointment 6%
d. Crotamiton 10%

10. Which of the following statements regarding treatment of pediculosis capitis is true?

   a. Carpeting and furniture should be shampooed and sprayed with a pediculocide. *vacuuming but not spraying*
   b. Nonwashable items should be sealed in plastic bags for 2 to 4 weeks
   c. Hair must be trimmed close to the scalp to insure elimination of nits *no*
   d. Frequent shampooing with Permethrin 1% will prevent reinfestation *no*

11. You note a single, large, oval pink patch with central clearing on 16-year-old M.P.'s back. Lesions are not present elsewhere. Results of a KOH preperation of the lesion are negative. This would confirm a diagnosis of:

   a. Seborrheic dermatitis
   b. Secondary syphilis
   c. Tinea corporis *⊕ KOH*
   d. Pityriasis rosea

12. Mrs. J. brings her 6-year-old son in because of "hives" that she describes as a red raised rash. Which finding below would support a diagnosis of erythema multiforme rather than urticaria?

   a. Lesions that blanch with pressure
   b. Eyelid edema
   c. Lesions that are present for more than 24 hours *(erythema multiforme)*
   d. Intense itching

13. When examining 7-month-old R.V. you note red scaly plaques in his diaper area, particularly in the inguinal folds, with satellite lesions on his abdomen. The appropriate treatment would be:

   a. Petrolatum/lanolin ointment
   b. Petroleum jelley   *} barrier products*
   c. Zinc oxide
   d. Nystatin *candida*

Questions 14 and 15 refer to the following scenario.

During 15-year-old N.M.'s routine physical examination she complains of getting pimples all the time. You note open and closed comedones over her forehead and chin. There are several pustules but no cysts.

14. Which of the medications below is the appropriate choice?

    a. Oral contraceptives
    b. Isotretinoin
    c. Tetracycline
    d. Etretinate

15. Which of the following should N.M. avoid when using the medication in the above question?

    a. Oil based cosmetics
    b. Vitamin A supplements
    c. Alcohol
    d. Dairy products

16. Which of the following statements is not consistent with an appropriate management plan for acne?

    a. Improvement with use of keratolytic agents should occur within 4 to 6 weeks
    b. Facial scrubs are recommended before applying topical antibiotics
    e. Noncomedogenic moisturizers and cosmetics may be used
    d. Sunscreens should always be used in conjunction with retinoic acid

17. H.B. is 2-days-old. Her mother calls and reports a rash consisting of redness with yellow-white "bumps" all over her body except for the palms and soles. The infant most likely has:

    a. Erythema toxicum
    b. Transient neonatal pustular melanosis
    c. Molluscum contagiosum
    d. Milia

Questions 18 and 19 refer to the following scenario.

6-year-old L.R. presents at clinic with a single weepy lesion around his upper lip. Closer inspection reveals some vesicles and honey colored crusts.

18. The most likely diagnosis is:

    a. Herpes simplex

b. Varicella

c. Nummular eczema

d. Impetigo

19. The treatment of choice for L.R. would be:

a. Acyclovir

b. Topical steroids

c. Topical antibiotics   *mupirocin (bactroban)*

d. Petrolatum/lanolin ointment

20. D.J. is a 4-year-old African-American child with a depigmented patch on his forehead. The lesion has sharp borders. No scales are present. The most appropriate treatment would be:

a. 1% hydrocortisone   *vitiligo responds to steroids 30-50% of the time*

b. Alpha hydroxy acid

c. Ketoconazole

d. Silver sulfadiazine

21. While examining 7-year-old S.R.'s scalp you note three small patches of hair loss. Broken hair is present as is erythema and scaling. Based on this information, which of the following diagnoses is most likely?

a. Tinea capitis

b. Traction alopecia

c. Trichotillomania

d. Alopecia areata

Answers and Rationale

1. **(c)** Common warts are found most usually on fingers, hands and feet in children, and are often preceded by trauma such as nail biting or picking at cuticles (Zitelli & Davis, p. 242).

2. **(b)** Striae describes skin that has been stretched, whereas the skin in atopic dermatitis is thickened, crusted, and hyperpigmented (Burns, et al., p. 505, 740).

3. **(a)** The infantile phase of atopic dermatitis follows a different distribution pattern then that associated with the childhood phase which may include the face, trunk, and extensor surfaces (Zitelli & Davis, pp. 217-218).

4. **(d)** While all of the choices have a bluish discoloration, cutis marmorata is the only condition that is generalized (Burns, et al., p. 805).

5. **(c)** The lesions described are café au lait spots. Six or more of these lesions may indicate neurofibromatosis and should be referred for further evaluation (Burns, et al., p. 764).

6. **(b)** A salmon patch is a flat, light pink to light red mark seen on the eyelid, glabella, or nape of neck that intensifies with crying (Fox, p. 580).

7. **(a)** The rash described is *Candida albicans* and should be treated with an antifungal agent (Fox, p. 597).

8. **(b)** Microscopic skin scrapings of burrows will reveal the mite, eggs, or feces if scabies are present. Although skin scrapings are not routinely done, they are definitive if there is any doubt of the diagnosis (Burns, et al., p. 758).

9. **(a)** Permethrin is the only safe choice in this case. Lindane is contraindicated in infants under six months. Sulfur ointment and crotamiton are not as effective and are difficult to use (Burns, et al., p. 759).

10. **(b)** Objects which cannot be washed should be sealed in plastic bags. Since eggs mature in 7 to 10 days, 2 to 4 weeks should be sufficient to prevent

reinfestation. Frequent shampooing and close haircuts are unnecessary and may contribute to a feeling of shame and embarrassment. Environmental cleaning includes vacuuming, and sprays are not recommended (Burns, et al., p. 758).

11. **(d)** Pityriasis rosea presents with a herald patch, is probably viral, and thus will not reveal hyphae or spores seen in the KOH scrapings of fungal infections such as tinea. The location of the patch and its absence on the mucosa, palms, and soles distinguish it from seborrheic dermatitis and secondary syphilis (Zitelli & Davis, pp. 200-222).

12. **(c)** Urticarial lesions tend to be pruritic and blanch with pressure but generally fade within a few hours. Due to the large number of mast cells present in the eyelids, edema is common with urticaria. The lesions of erythema multiforme are fixed and present for up to 2 to 3 weeks (Gartner & Zitelli, p. 318).

13. **(d)** Answers "a," "b," and "c" are all ointments which act as barriers to irritants such as urine and feces. The presence of satellite lesions indicate a candida rash requiring an antifungal such as nystatin (Zitelli & Davis, p. 223).

14. **(c)** Moderate acne includes open and closed comedones, papules, and pustules. Oral antibiotics are used to control moderate papulopustular acne in addition to topical keratolytics. Oral contraceptives and antiandrogens are used when other therapies have been unsuccessful. Etretinate is a retinoic acid used in the treatment of psoriasis. Isotretinoin is a vitamin A derivative used only in the most recalcitrant of cases (Burns, et al., p. 577; Fox, p. 752; Ellsworth, et al., pp. 341, 454).

15. **(d)** Occlusive cosmetics can contribute to the problem by plugging the follicular duct. Absorption of tetracycline is decreased when taken with dairy products. Vitamin A and alcohol should be avoided when taking etretinate or isotretinoin because of Vitamin A toxicity and hepatotoxicity respectively (Ellsworth, et al., pp. 341, 454; Fox, p. 577).

16. **(b)** Facial scrubs are not recommended and may exacerbate acne (Fox, p. 579; Burns, et al., p. 752).

17. **(a)** The location (all over the body) and type of lesion (papule as opposed to vesicle) are consistent with the rash seen in erythema toxicum (Hoekelman et al., p. 527).

18. **(d)** The classic presentation of impetigo is that of vesicles that rupture leaving honey colored crusts (Burns, et al., p. 745)

19. **(c)** Impetigo is a bacterial infection, most likely caused by *S. aureus*, group A β-hemolytic streptococcus, or *Streptococcus pyogenes*. Mild cases may be treated with topical antibiotics; if no resolution, systemic antibiotics may be necessary (Burns, et al., 745)

20. **(a)** The most likely diagnosis is vitiligo, an area of depigmented skin more common in people of color. It responds to steroids 30% to 50% of the time. Antifungals, antibiotics, or keratolytics would be of no value (Burns, et al., p. 765; Hoekelman, et al., p. 1201).

21. **(a)** Erythema, scaling, and broken hair are characteristic findings associated with tinea capitis. Traction alopecia may have associated erythema but not scaling. While neither trichotillomania or alopecia areata are associated with erythema or scaling, only alopecia areata is noted for total hair loss (Burns, et al., pp. 765-766; Zitelli & Davis, pp. 258, 260).

References

Burns, C. E., Barber, N., Brady, M. A., & Dunn, A. M. (Eds.). (1996). *Pediatric primary care: A handbook for nurse practitioners.* Philadelphia: W. B. Saunders.

Fox, J. A. (Ed.). (1997). *Primary health care of children.* St. Louis: Mosby.

Ellsworth, A. J., Witt, D. M., Dugdale, D. C., & Oliver, L. M. (Eds.). (1998). *1998 Medical drug reference.* St. Louis: Mosby.

Gartner, J. C., & Zitelli, B. J. (Ed.). (1997). *Common and chronic symptoms in pediatrics.* St. Louis: Mosby.

Hoekelman, R. A., Friedman, S. B., Nelson, N. M., Seidel, H. M., & Weitzman, M. L. (Eds.). (1997). *Primary pediatric care.* St. Louis: Mosby.

Zitelli, B. J., & Davis, H. W. (Eds.). (1997). *Atlas of pediatric physical diagnosis* (3rd ed.). St. Louis: Mosby.

Note: This chapter was written by Patricia Clinton prior to her appointment as certification chair representing the National Association of Pediatric Nurse Associates and Practitioners (NAPNAP) to the National Certification Board of Pediatric Nurse Practitioners and Nurses.

Gastrointestinal Disorders

Patricia Clinton

Select one best answer to the following questions.

Questions 1 and 2 refer to the following scenario.

The mother of 4-month-old N.D. reports episodes of vomiting and diarrhea beginning two days ago. He has also had several episodes of screaming and drawing up his legs. Prior to this he has been healthy with a normal weight gain.

1. The least likely diagnosis is:

    a. Incarcerated hernia
    b. Gastroenteritis
    c. Intussusception
    d. Pyloric stenosis

2. Physical examination of N.D. reveals a sausage shaped mass and guaiac positive stool. This would confirm a diagnosis of:

    a. Incarcerated hernia
    b. Gastroenteritis
    c. Intussusception
    d. Pyloric stenosis

3. 14-year-old R.D. presents with a complaint of abdominal pain that has occurred several times over the past three months. She describes the pain as an intermittent sharp pain, occasionally relieved with a heating pad. Her physical examination is within normal limits. You suspect recurrent abdominal pain (RAP). Which clinical finding is most consistent with RAP?

    a. Periumbilical pain
    b. Constipation
    c. Pain worsens with defecation
    d. Weight loss

4. Education and counseling of the parents of a 4-month-old child with gastro-esophageal reflux should include which of the following?

    a. Place infant on left side after eating *prone pc*

    b. Change to a hypoallergenic formula

    c. Place infant in a swing after feeding

    d. Decrease volume and increase frequency of feedings

5. 6-year-old B.W. complains of sharp epigastric pain radiating to his back. Which laboratory data would be consistent with these physical signs?

    a. Decreased serum albumin

    b. Elevated serum amylase *- pancreatitis*

    c. Elevated serum gastrin

    d. Decreased serum protein

6. An umbilical hernia:

    a. Occurs more frequently in full term infants

    b. Resolves spontaneously in 3 to 6 months

    c. Is frequently associated with diastasis recti

    d. Responds well to taping

7. 9-year-old S.L. is brought to the clinic for evaluation of abdominal pain that wakes her at night. Her parents have recently divorced and she is attending a new school. She has missed eight days of school in the past six weeks. She reports occasional emesis. An appropriate management plan would be:

    a. A bland diet with small frequent feedings

    b. A referral to a pediatrician *PUD*

    c. To stress importance of school attendance

    d. To consult with the school psychologist

Questions 8 and 9 refer to the following scenario.

7-month-old J.D. is seen with a two day history of diarrhea. He has had 3 to 4 wet diapers in the past 24 hours. The anterior fontanel is slightly depressed. Capillary refill is normal.

8. Which degree of dehydration is most consistent with these findings?

    a. 4%

    b. 5%

mild 3-5
mod. 6-9
sev. ≥10

c. 8%
d. 10%

9. Based on your assessment of J.D., the appropriate management plan for his de-hydration would be to:

    a. Begin BRAT diet
    b. Withhold formula for 24 hours and give electrolyte solution
    c. Begin rehydration in the office and observe for 3 to 4 hours
    d. Refer immediately for parenteral fluids

10. 3-day-old A.W. presents with vomiting, abdominal distention, and constipation. Which of the following should be included in the differential diagnosis?

    a. Hirschsprung disease
    b. Pyloric stenosis
    c. Celiac disease
    d. Meckel diverticulum

11. 4-year-old C.R. was diagnosed with celiac disease at age 18 months. In addi-tion to closely monitoring her growth you also monitor for anemia. At this visit her laboratory results confirm an elevated MCV. An appropriate follow-up labo-ratory test would be serum:

    a. Protein
    b. Ferritin ↓ mcv
    c. Folate
    d. Transferrin

↑ mcv = macrocytosis = ↓ folate

— celiac dz assoc c̄ folic acid deficiency

(↓ mcv and ↑ RDW = ↓ Fe (hgb))

12. 11-year-old Justin presents with complaints of chronic diarrhea and abdominal pain. You note a 5 kg weight loss from last year's annual examination. Today his examination reveals right lower quadrant pain and perianal skin tags. The most likely diagnosis is:

    a. Encoporesis
    b. Crohn's disease
    c. Irritable bowel disease
    d. Ulcerative colitis

Questions 13 and 14 refer to the following scenario.

9-year-old E.G. presents with diffuse abdominal pain and acute onset of diarrhea described as a frequent urge to defecate. She is passing large amounts of flatus, small amounts of stool, and complains of tenderness during rectal examination.

13. This clinical picture is highly suggestive of:

    a. Gastroenteritis
    b. Ulcerative colitis
    c. Giardiasis
    d. Appendicitis

14. Which of the following laboratory tests would confirm your diagnosis for E.G.?

    a. Serum albumin *no*
    b. Abdominal ultrasound
    c. Stool for ova and parasites *no*
    d. Bone age *no*

15. After returning from a three week family vacation, Mrs. K. learns that the day care her 7-month-old daughter Jessica will be attending has had a recent outbreak of hepatitis A. Before taking Jessica to the day care Mrs. K. asks your advice. You would suggest:

    a. Reviewing diaper changing policy with day care staff
    b. Immunizing with hepatitis A virus vaccine *not < 2yoa*
    c. Administering immune globulin IM *post-exposure only*
    d. Waiting two weeks before sending her to day care *not necessary*

16. 7-year-old J.V. presents with a one week history of fever, nausea, and anorexia. His mother reports that his skin "looks funny" as well. Further laboratory studies confirm a diagnosis of viral hepatitis. Which type of hepatitis is the most likely?

    a. Hepatitis A   *fever common c̄ HAV*
    b. Hepatitis B
    c. Hepatitis C
    d. Hepatitis D

17. 2-week-old C.A. is being seen for the first time since discharge from the newborn nursery. She currently weighs 3.6 kg which is 0.3 kg below her birth weight. While interviewing her mother you learn she has been using too little

water when preparing the formula. Which of the following symptoms would not likely be related to this error?

   a. Vomiting ✓
   b. Diarrhea ✓
   c. Dehydration ✓
   d. Flatus — *usually 2° swallowing too much air*

18. Vomitus that is bilious suggests:

   a. GI obstruction proximal to the pylorus *no*
   b. GI obstruction below the ampulla of Vater *(hepatopancreatic)*
   c. Pyloric stenosis *no*
   d. Peptic ulcer disease *no*

19. 5-year-old J.P. presents with a history of stool staining his underwear, evidence of bright red blood after wiping, and abdominal discomfort. The physical examination reveals moderate abdominal distension with a midline abdominal mass. Rectal examination is positive for an impacted rectum and two small anal fissures. The priority in your management plan would be:

   a. Increasing water and fiber in the diet, limiting milk intake
   b. Regular toilet sitting for 10 minutes three times per day
   c. Two fleet enemas *to remove impaction*
   d. Mineral oil after breakfast and before bed

20. Which of the following would not be included in the management of pinworms?

   a. Nutritional support and iron supplementation
   b. Simultaneous treatment of all family members ✓
   c. Washing bed linen in hot water ✓
   d. Keeping fingernails short and clean ✓

21. Mrs. D. reports starting her 6-month-old infant on rice cereal sweetened with one tablespoon of honey. In addition the infant is consuming 42 ounces of formula. His height and weight are at 50% on the growth curve. You would recommend:

   a. Adding pureed vegetables
   b. Substituting 4 oz. juice for a formula feeding
   c. Adding scrambled egg whites
   d. Discontinuing honey *2° potential infection c̄ clostridium botulinum*

Answers and Rationale

1 **(d)** Pyloric stenosis occurs during the first few weeks of life with projectile vomiting and weight loss (Burns, et al., pp. 669, 811).

2. **(c)** Invagination of the bowel can result in a sausage like mass being palpated in the upper right quadrant of the abdomen with occasional bloody stools (Burns, et al., p. 669).

3. **(a)** Recurrent abdominal pain is almost always nonorganic in origin. Other than complaints of pain, usually periumbilical or midepigastric, the history and physical examination are normal (Fox, p. 792; Burns, et al., p. 670).

4. **(d)** The purpose of small frequent feedings is to lessen the abdominal distention. Formula changes are controversial and probably make little difference. Infant swings will worsen symptoms by increasing intra-abdominal pressure. The infant should be placed in the prone position for 1 to 2 hours after feeding (Fox, p. 528-529).

5. **(b)** The physical signs described are characteristic of pancreatitis which can be confirmed with a serum amylase. Decreased serum albumin and protein are associated with Crohn's disease. The clinical picture of Crohn's disease usually includes cramping and does not radiate to the back (Fox, p. 482).

6. **(c)** Umbilical hernias are a result of incomplete closure of the fascia of the umbilical ring which, if small, may close by one year. The incidence is higher in low birth weight and premature infants. There is no evidence that manual reduction such as taping hastens closure (Burns, et al., p. 813; Behrman, 441; Fox, p. 502).

7. **(b)** Initially because of the social history, one might think that this recurrent abdominal pain is part of school refusal syndrome. However, the night waking and occasional emesis suggests peptic ulcer disease. Changes in diet are not usually effective in treating peptic ulcers. This warrants immediate referral to a pediatrician (Burns, et al., p. 668; Fox, p. 480; Zitelli & Davis, p. 295).

8. **(c)** A depressed fontanel and decreased urinary output are indicative of moderate (8%) dehydration (Hoekelman, et al., p. 1668).

9. **(c)** The appropriate treatment for moderate dehydration is oral rehydration begun at the health care setting and observation until the rehydration phase is completed (Hoekelman, et al., p. 1669).

10. **(a)** Age and clinical findings are helpful in establishing this diagnosis. Celiac disease presents with diarrhea. Pyloric stenosis is not associated with abdominal distention, and Meckel diverticulum presents in the toddler period as painless rectal bleeding. Hirschsprung should be suspected in any newborn with abdominal distention and difficulty passing stool (Fox, pp. 536-537; Behrman, et al., p. 442).

11. **(c)** Celiac disease is frequently associated with folic acid deficiency. An elevated MCV indicates macrocytosis. Anemia due to folate deficiency is macrocytic (Burns, et al., pp. 538-539).

12. **(b)** While abdominal pain and diarrhea are common to all the choices, the right lower quadrant pain is more suggestive of Crohn's disease. Perianal skin tags are common in Crohn's disease but would be unlikely in the others (Burns, et al., p.671)

13. **(d)** Large amounts of gas and watery stools occur about 15% of the time in appendicitis and pain upon rectal examination is a classic symptom (Burns, et al., p. 668).

14. **(b)** Abdominal ultrasound can reveal an enlarged appendix and help to eliminate ovarian or pelvic disease. Serum albumin and ESR would be useful in diagnosing ulcerative colitis. Stool for O & P would be diagnostic of giardiasis (Behrman, et al., p. 420-421).

15. **(a)** Hepatitis A is transmitted through the fecal-oral route and can be prevented with proper sanitation and good hygiene practices. HAV vaccine is not approved for children less than two years old. Immune globulin is recommended within two weeks after exposure (which this infant was not). The highest period of contagion is 1 to 2 weeks prior to onset of symptoms, so

the infant would not benefit from staying home at this time (AAP, pp. 237-238).

16. **(a)** The acute onset and presence of fever as well as jaundice is associated with hepatitis A. Fevers are less common with the other viral hepatitis conditions (Hoekelman, et al., p. 1339).

17. **(d)** Vomiting in the newborn period may be caused by improper preparation of formula. Too little water will increase the GI and renal solute load which may result in vomiting, diarrhea and dehydration. Flatus is usually a result of swallowing too much air (Gartner & Zitelli, p. 277).

18. **(b)** Vomiting bile is generally considered a serious sign that usually indicates an obstruction below the ampulla of Vater (Hoekelman, et al., p. 1152).

19. **(c)** The clinical picture is consistent with encoporesis. The abdomen can be distended and often a mass is palpated. Anal fissures may be present from straining but skin tags are unlikely. The first step in treatment is to remove the impaction. Once the colon is cleared, maintenance with stool softeners, diet, and regular toileting is appropriate (Burns, et al., p. 284; Hoekelman, et al., p. 722).

20. **(a)** Pinworms are a common parasite infecting children. They are easily treated with medication and simple environmental measures. No nutritional deficiencies are associated with pinworms (Burns, et al., p. 678; Fox, p. 532).

21. **(d)** Honey may contain *C. botulinum* spores and should not be given to infants less than one year old. Adding vegetables is appropriate, but the risk of infant botulism is potentially life threatening. Although juice may be added it should not be substituted for formula. Egg whites may be added at the end of the first year (AAP, p. 175; Behrman, et al., p. 351-352; Kleinman p. 47).

References

American Academy of Pediatrics (AAP). (1997). *Redbook: Report of the committee on infectious diseases* (24th ed.). Elk Grove Village, IL: Author.

Behrman, R. E., & Kliegman, R. M. (Ed.). (1998). *Nelson essentials of pediatrics* (3rd ed.). Philadelphia: W. B. Saunders.

Burns, C. E., Barber, N., Brady, M.A., & Dunn, A. M. (Eds.). (1996). *Pediatric primary care: A handbook for nurse practitioners.* Philadelphia: W. B. Saunders.

Fox, J. A. (Ed.). (1997). *Primary health care of children.* St. Louis: Mosby.

Gartner, J. C., & Zitelli, B. J. (Eds.). (1997). *Common and chronic symptoms in pediatrics.* St. Louis: Mosby.

Hoekelman, R. A., Friedman, S. B., Nelson, N. M., Seidel, H. M., & Weitzman, M. L. (Eds.). (1997). *Primary pediatric care.* St. Louis: Mosby.

Kleinman, R. E. (Ed.). (1998). *Pediatric nutrition handbook* (4th ed.). Elk Grove Village, IL: American Academy of Pediatrics.

Zitelli, B. J., & Davis, H. W. (Eds). (1997). *Atlas of pediatric physical diagnosis* (3rd ed.). St. Louis: Mosby.

Note: This chapter was written by Patricia Clinton prior to her appointment as certification chair representing the National Association of Pediatric Nurse Associates and Practitioners (NAPNAP) to the National Certification Board of Pediatric Nurse Practitioners and Nurses.

Infectious Diseases

Brenda Holloway

Select one best answer to the following questions.

1. Sam's mother has telephoned the clinic because chickenpox has been "going around" at Sam's school and she has just noticed a few red spots along the hairline on his face. She asks if there is anything that can be given to shorten the duration or severity of the illness. Which answer is appropriate?

   a. Diphenhydramine elixir has been shown to shorten the duration and severity of the rash
   b. Acyclovir has been shown to shorten the duration and severity of the illness
   c. Aspirin taken four times a day has been shown to shorten the duration and severity of the illness
   d. There is no medication known to alter the course of the illness

2. A 14-year-old has been diagnosed with mononucleosis. The PNP should teach the adolescent and the parents that which of the following should be avoided?

   a. Strenuous exercise if the spleen is palpable
   b. Weight bearing activities until laboratory tests show resolution of the disease
   c. Unnecessary activity until lymph nodes return to normal size
   d. Stretching and reaching activities during the acute stage of illness

3. A well nourished 10-year-old female presents to the clinic with low grade fever, sore throat, fatigue and malaise, and left upper abdominal pain. Based on clinical presentation and laboratory results, a diagnosis of infectious mononucleosis is made. Which of the presenting signs and symptoms requires further investigation immediately?

   a. Low grade fever
   b. Sore throat with lymphadenopathy
   c. Fatigue and malaise

(d.) Left upper abdominal pain

4. Initial treatment for a child with uncomplicated infectious mononucleosis should include:

   a. Home care with bed rest progressing to activity as tolerated
   b. Home care with complete bedrest until afebrile
   c. Hospitalization with complete bedrest until laboratory values return to normal
   d. Hospitalization with daily, planned physical therapy

5. You are performing a physical examination on a 12-year-old boy who is planning to go to summer camp in a primitive wooded area. What teaching is appropriate for the prevention of Rocky Mountain spotted fever?

   a. Inspect the body several times a day and remove ticks immediately
   b. Inspect the skin while taking a shower and apply soap to ticks before removing
   c. Ticks should be removed only after they have been killed with alcohol
   d. Tick removal should be performed by a health care professional

6. 4-day-old Kali has been brought to the clinic because her eyes have been draining. Conjunctival culture reveals *Chlamydia trachomatis* as the cause. Appropriate treatment is:

   a. Tetracycline eye ointment
   b. Oral erythromycin
   c. Intramuscular penicillin
   d. Intravenous gentamycin

Questions 7, 8, and 9 refer to the following scenario.

8-year-old John's mother telephones to tell you that John developed chickenpox three days ago. She wants to know if there is anything she can do to make him more comfortable.

7. You should tell John's mother to:

   a. Apply topical calamine lotion
   b. Apply a topical antibiotic to the new vesicles
   c. Give aspirin for fever and discomfort
   d. Keep John out of bright light

8. You should also tell John's mother to:

   a. Avoid getting the lesions wet
   b. Encourage John to take a bath everyday
   c. Have John take a bath only if he develops fever and sweats
   d. Encourage John to take only sponge baths until all lesions are healed

9. Ten days after onset of the initial rash, John's mother calls you again to report that John has had a severe headache since yesterday and that he is very irritable. You should:

   a. Ask the mother if John has had a bowel movement since he has been ill
   b. Tell John's mother that these symptoms are common when chickenpox is resolving
   c. Ask the mother if there is a family history of severe headaches
   d. Ask John's mother to bring him to the office today for evaluation

10. A 16-year-old male has been diagnosed with measles (rubeola). He is also complaining of ear pain. His tympanic membranes are red and bulging. Appropriate management of the ear problem is to treat the ears with:

    a. Pain medication until the virus has run its course
    b. The same medication used to treat any case of otitis media
    c. Liquid topical antibiotics and topical steroids
    d. Acyclovir given by mouth

11. Seven-year-old Bob's mother has brought him to the clinic because he has a rash. Physical examination reveals vesicles on the hands, feet, and in the mouth. Hand-foot and mouth disease is diagnosed. Treatment is based on:

    a. Alleviating symptoms
    b. Eradication of causative bacteria
    c. Prevention of febrile convulsions
    d. Prevention of secondary infections

12. Six-year-old Cali's mother brings her to the clinic because the family is planning a trip to a tropical area, and she wants to know how to avoid illness. Knowing that cases of malaria have been reported in the area, you should teach:

    a. Avoidance of contact with infected people
    b. Hand washing after touching contaminated fomites
    c. Avoidance of mosquito bites
    d. Cooking of all vegetables

13. Six-year-old Steven has been diagnosed with erythema infectiosum (fifth disease). His mother asks you how to prevent spread of the disease to her other children. Your answer should be that:

    a. The disease is not thought to be contagious
    b. Stephen should eat and drink from disposable containers
    c. Other children should not be allowed to touch the erythematous areas
    d. By the time the rash appears, the patient is no longer contagious

14. Considering the pathophysiology associated with erythema infectiosum (fifth disease), which child with the disease must be monitored closely? The child who has a history of:

    a. Frequent respiratory infections
    b. Multiple skin allergies
    c. Malabsorption syndrome
    d. Hemolytic anemia

15. Four-day-old Susan's mother has brought her to the clinic because she hasn't seemed interested in her bottle since yesterday. Physical examination reveals a lethargic infant with an axillary temperature of 96° F and a pulse rate of 100. Extremities are slightly cool. Appropriate management includes:

    a. Reassuring the mother that infants tend to regulate their own feeding habits
    b. Instructing the mother on proper nipple placement and feeding techniques
    c. Changing the infant to a soy based formula and re-evaluating her in 24 hours
    d. Referring the infant to a pediatrician for further evaluation   ? sepsis

16. The mother of a toddler with a typical roseola type rash and a history of high fever asks if there is any treatment available for the condition. The PNP tells the mother that:

    a. Topical corticosteroids are helpful to relieve itching
    b. Oral diphenhydramine is helpful to decrease desquamation
    c. Aspirin should be used to treat the typical high fever
    d. There is no medical treatment for roseola

17. Mrs. Chancellor contracted rubella while pregnant with 1-month-old Andrew. Andrew should be considered contagious for what time period?

    a. Five to 7 days
    b. Until he is afebrile

c. At least the first year of life
d. He is not contagious

18. Four-year-old James has been diagnosed with cat scratch disease. His mother asks what should be done about the cat. Your response should be that:

a. The cat should be isolated until it can be treated with antibiotics
b. The cat should be isolated until it can be treated with antihelmintics
c. The cat should be evaluated by a medical laboratory and destroyed
d. There are no recommendations for treating or destroying the cat

19. Which of the following vaccines is contraindicated for routine use in a 3-year-old who is receiving vincristine for maintenance treatment of acute lymphocytic leukemia?

a. DPT
b. Influenza
c. MMR — *live virus*
d. Hepatitis B

20. Eight-year-old Grant has been home schooled for the past two years. His mother now plans to enroll him in public school and has brought him to the clinic because the school officials have told her that his immunizations must be updated. Which of the following immunizations should not be given to Grant?

a. Diphtheria
b. Pertussis
c. Tetanus
d. Tetanus diphtheria combination

21. One-year-old Stephanie is infected with HIV. When should her MMR immunization be given?

a. According to the usual schedule
b. Only when the CD4+ count is at a safe level
c. Only if she attends day care
d. MMR should not be given to Stephanie

22. A 15-year-old with immunodeficiency disease has come to the clinic for an immunization update. His record shows he has received only two doses of IPV. Which action is appropriate?

a. Give a dose of IPV
b. Give a dose of OPV

    c. Give no polio vaccine now

    d. Refer him to an infectious disease specialist

23. When a child is given IPV rather than OPV, what teaching is necessary?

    a. The schedule and dosing are the same for both IPV and OPV no

    b. IPV should not be given if the child will be around anyone who is pregnant no

    c. IPV should not be given to any child who is allergic to bee venom no

    d. Booster doses of IPV may be needed after age 6

Answers and Rationale

1. **(b)** Acyclovir has been shown to slightly shorten the duration of fever and new lesion formation. Aspirin is not given to children with chickenpox because of it's association with Reye's syndrome (Oski, et al., pp. 1335-1336).

2. **(a)** To avoid splenic rupture, strenuous exercise and contact sports should be avoided as long as the spleen is palpable (Hoekelman, et al., p. 1372).

3. **(d)** Left upper abdominal pain should alert the practitioner to the possibility of splenic rupture. Sore throat should be cultured for strep if this has not been done (strep is a differential diagnosis for this presentation and strep often co-exists with mono) but the need for the culture is not urgent (Hoekelman, et al., pp. 1371-1372).

4. **(a)** Bedrest and activity as tolerated are recommended in the initial treatment of uncomplicated infectious mononucleosis (Oski, et al., p. 1318).

5. **(a)** Ticks must be attached for 4 to 6 hours or more before they can transmit Rocky Mountain spotted fever; frequent removal of ticks is valuable. Ticks do not need to be treated with soap or alcohol before removal, and do not need to be removed by a health care provider (Oski, et al., p. 1362).

6. **(b)** Oral erythromycin is the treatment of choice. Eye drops or ointments are not effective for the prevention or treatment of neonatal chlamydial conjunctivitis. Intramuscular and intravenous antibiotics are not needed (Oski, et al., p. 1357).

7. **(a)** Itching causes discomfort in children with chickenpox. Calamine lotion may be applied liberally for relief of itching caused by vesicular lesions. Neosporin does not decrease itching. Steroids may weaken the immune system and should not be used on the child with a herpes virus. Photophobia frequently occurs in rubeola (measles) but not chickenpox (Oski, et al., p. 1335).

8. **(b)** There are no restrictions on bathing. Children with chickenpox should be encouraged to take daily baths to help prevent secondary bacterial infection

which is the most common complication of chickenpox (Hoekelman, et al., p. 1240).

9. **(d)** Cerebellar complications or cerebral infections may occur as a complication associated with chickenpox. These complications may occur four days preceding the rash until three weeks after the appearance of the rash. John's headache and irritability are signs that there may be an encephalopathy. John should be evaluated in the office to rule out this possibility (Hoekelman, et al., p. 1240).

10. **(b)** Otitis media is common with measles. It is treated as any acute otitis media (Hoekelman, et al., p. 1264).

11. **(a)** The course of hand-foot and mouth disease (thought to be caused by a coxsackievirus) is usually benign and treatment is symptomatic. Fever is usually low grade and the throat is sore (Hoekelman, et al., pp. 1296; Oski, et al., p. 915).

12. **(c)** The malaria parasite is spread by the mosquito's bite (Hoekelman, et al., p. 1478).

13. **(d)** Erythema infectiosum is only contagious before the rash appears. The mode of transmission is unclear (Oski, et al., p. 1304).

14. **(d)** The profound reticulocytopenia associated with erythema contagiosum may result in a dangerous decrease of hemoglobin concentration in the child with hemolytic anemias such as sickle cell or thalassemia, pyruvate kinase deficiency, or acquired hemolytic anemias (Oski, et al., p. 1304).

15. **(d)** The neonate with sepsis often presents with hypothermia, lethargy, poor feeding, and bradycardia. The infant should be referred to a pediatrician for a sepsis evaluation (Oski. et al., pp. 385, 518, 1119).

16. **(d)** There is no medical treatment for roseola. Febrile seizure is the most common complication of roseola, but the appearance of the diagnostic rash usually coincides with the abrupt termination of fever. Itching and desquamation are not associated with roseola (Oski, et al., pp. 1330-1331).

17. **(c)** Infants with congenital rubella may excrete the virus from the nasopharynx and in the urine for a year (Oski, et al., p. 1338).

18. **(d)** The capacity for disease transmission by cats appears to be transient. There are no recommendations for treating or destroying the cat. The cat may be declawed but the disease can also be induced by cat bites (Oski, et al., p. 1421).

19. **(c)** MMR contains live virus vaccine and should not be given to a child (without consultation with a specialist) who is on immunosuppressive therapy, including chemotherapeutic agents such as vincristine (Oski, et al., p. 1339).

20. **(b)** Pertussis immunization is not given routinely to children over age seven years because severe pertussis is a disease of young children and reaction to immunization appears to increase with age (Oski, et al., p. 1211).

21. **(a)** Live virus is generally not given to immunodeficient children. The exception is children infected with HIV, who should be immunized against MMR at the appropriate age (CDC, pp. 8-12).

22. **(a)** OPV contains live virus and is not given to the immunodeficient child. IPV, the inactivated immunization, is used instead (CDC, pp. 8-12).

23. **(d)** IPV (the inactivated parenterally administered polio virus vaccine) produces a lesser degree of immunity than OPV and, though it is uncertain, booster doses may be needed every five years (CDC, pp. 8-12).

References

Centers for Disease Control and Prevention. (1998). Recommended childhood immunization schedule. *Morbidity and Mortality Weekly Report, 47*(01), 8-12.

Hoekelman, R. A., Friedman, S. B., Nelson, N. M., Seidel, H. M., & Weitzman, M. L. (Eds.). (1997). *Primary pediatric care* (3rd ed.). St. Louis: Mosby.

Jarvis, C. (1996). *Physical examination and health assessment.* Philadelphia: W. B. Saunders.

Oski, F. A., DeAngelis, C. D., Feigin, R. D., McMillan, J. A., & Warshaw, J. B. (Eds.). (1994). *Principles and practice of pediatrics.* Philadelphia: J. B. Lippincott.

Musculoskeletal Disorders

Patricia Clinton

Select one best answer to the following questions.

1. An injury at which of the following sites will most likely result in a length discrepancy?

   a. Diaphysis
   b. Epiphysis
   c. Medullary cavity
   d. Metaphysis

2. Growth in muscle length is related to:

   a. Growth in length of underlying bone
   b. Growth in length of underlying ligament
   c. Growth in length of underlying tendon
   d. Growth in length of opposing muscle group

3. Varus between the tibia and femur of up to 15° followed by a progression to a neutral angle which then progresses to valgus between 7° to 9° is associated with:

   a. Blount disease
   b. Internal tibial torsion
   c. Normal developmental growth pattern
   d. Abnormal tibiofemoral growth pattern

4. 8-year-old Tracy complains that she doesn't like to wear shorts because her knees look funny. Upon examination you note a genu valgum angle of greater than 15°. You should:

   a. Re-evaluate in one year
   b. Consult with a pediatrician
   c. Instruct her to avoid the "W" sitting position

    d. Encourage exercise to strengthen quadriceps

5. The appropriate treatment for genu varum in a 15-month-old is:

    a. Passive exercise with each diaper change
    b. Denis Browne splint at night
    c. Blount brace at night
    d. No treatment is warranted

6. During examination of 2-week-old J.P., you note irritability when lifted, asymmetrical Moro reflex, and spasm along the right sternocleidomastoid. This is most suggestive of:

    a. Torticollis
    b. Sprengel deformity
    c. Fractured clavicle
    d. Klippel-Feil syndrome

7. A child with growing pains is most likely to experience:

    a. A mild limp
    b. Bilateral lower extremity pain
    c. Lower extremity pain primarily during the day
    d. Lower extremity pain associated with decreased range of motion

8. 20-month-old C.W. presents in the emergency room with a greenstick fracture of his left femur. Physical examination also reveals an enlarged anterior fontanel and enlarged costochondral junction. These clinical findings suggest:

    a. Child abuse
    b. Osteogenesis imperfecta → fx's
    c. Osteoperosis
    d. Rickets

9. Which of the following represents appropriate anticipatory guidance for a child diagnosed with slipped capital femoral epiphysis?

    a. Avoid contact sports until growth is completed
    b. A wheelchair may facilitate mobility during acute phase
    c. Apply ice to affected area
    d. Range of motion and strengthening exercises

10. Which of the following findings would help distinguish slipped capital femoral epiphysis from Legg-Calve'-Perthes (LCP) disease?

a. Painful limp
b. Peak incidence at about seven years
c. Obesity
d. Antalgic limp

11. During 2½ year old Jason's physical examination you note large, muscular looking calves and observe difficulty rising from a sitting position. The Denver screening examination reveals delays in the gross motor area. Which of the following laboratory tests would be most beneficial?

    a. Serum calcium
    b. Serum magnesium
    c. Serum phosphorus
    d. Serum creatine kinase — *muscle function*

12. The appropriate management of Osgood-Schlatter's includes:

    a. Local injection of soluble corticosteroid
    b. Decrease activity, ice, NSAID
    c. Strengthening/stretching program for quadriceps
    d. Casting in adduction for six weeks

13. You have been treating 14-month-old J.V. for torticollis since birth. The condition has not resolved. The appropriate management plan would be to:

    a. Refer for surgical consultation
    b. Continue with passive range of motion
    c. Provide environmental stimulation opposite the contracture
    d. Apply cervical collar at night

14. While completing the hip examination on a newborn infant you are able to dislocate the infant's right hip. The appropriate management plan would be to:

    a. Triple diaper and re-evaluate in two weeks
    b. Recommend positioning prone while awake
    c. Refer to pediatrician
    d. Order tight swaddling of the infant

15. Which of the following would not be an appropriate test for developmental dysplasia of the hip in a 6-month-old child?

    a. Allis sign
    b. Skinfold symmetry
    c. Galeazzi sign

    d. Ortolani maneuver   *less reliable 2° diminished laxity*

16. 3-year-old T.C. presents with a history of fever for the past several days, pain in his left leg and refusal to bear weight on the left leg. Ten days ago he fell from a slide and bruised his leg. His WBC count is slightly elevated. You suspect either toxic synovitis or osteomyelitis. Which finding in this child supports a diagnosis of osteomyelitis rather than toxic synovitis?

    a. Recent injury
    b. Leg pain
    c. Nonweight bearing
    d. Elevated WBC

17. Which of the following suggests internal tibial torsion rather than internal femoral torsion in a 2-year-old child presenting with an in-toeing gait?

    a. Sitting in "W" position
    b. Knees face forward when walking
    c. Generalized ligament laxity
    d. Limited external rotation of hip

18. You examine C.J. in the newborn nursery and note a deformity in her left foot consisting of a convex lateral border and a forefoot which can be abducted past an imaginary line extending from the middle of the heel through the second toe. Which of the following management strategies is most appropriate?

    a. Reverse last shoes
    b. Out flare shoes
    c. Stretching exercises
    d. Orthopedic referral

19. A macular, salmon to red colored rash with irregular borders and central clearing is typical of:

    a. Systemic juvenile arthritis
    b. Lyme disease
    c. Systemic lupus erythematosus
    d. Rheumatic fever

20. 11-year-old L.J. presents with a nonpainful lateral curvature of the spine and waist asymmetry. Which of the following signs would be diagnostic of functional scoliosis?

    a. Positive Trendelenberg sign

    b. Negative Trendelenberg sign
    c. Positive Adam's sign
    (d.) Negative Adam's sign   "bend at the waist" exam

21. Coach Jones asks for advice on how to prevent "Little League" elbow in his 8 and 9 year old players. Which of the following would be incorrect advice?

    a. Have each child pitch only three innings ✓
    b. Limit or eliminate curve balls ✓
    (c.) Use ice massage before and after pitching   no
    d. Conduct slow warm-ups ✓

Answers and Rationale

1. **(b)** Bone length occurs at the epiphyseal plates which is also where the blood supply enters. If the blood supply is compromised growth is jeopardized (Burns, et al., p. 769).

2. **(a)** Growth in muscles is due to the range of motion the muscle is asked to perform as the underlying bone lengthens (Burns, et al., p. 770)

3. **(c)** The normal growth pattern is one of slight varus (bowleg) which progresses to a neutral angle and then slight valgus (knock-knee). Persistence of any phase beyond what is expected warrants further investigation (Burns, et al., p. 785).

4. **(b)** Valgus up to 15° is common up through the age of seven years, but persistence beyond that may lead to problems and degenerative changes and warrants referral (Behrman, et al., p. 756; Burns, et al., p. 784).

5. **(d)** Genu varum, or bowed leg, is normal until approximately 18 months (Burns, et al., p. 784).

6. **(c)** A fractured clavicle is not an uncommon finding following birth, especially in large babies. The spasm of the sternocleidomastoid and asymmetrical Moro reflex are classic signs of this problem (Burns, et al., p. 777).

7. **(b)** Growing pains tend to occur during rapid growth, increasing in prevalence after the age of 5. The pain is a muscular pain located bilaterally in the legs and thighs (Behrman, et al., p. 748; Fox, et al., p. 660).

8. **(d)** Rickets develops after several months of vitamin D deficiency and is characterized by craniotabes and enlarged anterior fontanel with delayed closing. The enlarged costochondral junction, or rachitic rosary, is a classic sign (Behrman, et al., p. 678).

9. **(a)** Treatment of slipped capital femoral epiphysis is aimed at preventing further slippage. Thus, the goal is no weight bearing and avoiding flexion of the hip as in wheelchair use. Once the growth plate closes contact sports

may be resumed. Ice would not change the problem in the femoral head and ROM and exercise are contraindicated (Burns, et al., p. 783; Fox, p. 655).

10. **(c)** A painful antalgic limp is common to both conditions. Obese preadolescent males are at risk for development of slipped capital femoral epiphysis (Burns, et al., p. 782; Fox, p. 651).

11. **(d)** Creatine kinase is an enzyme found in muscle and brain tissue and reflects tissue catabolism due to cell trauma. When muscle wasting occurs, as in muscular dystrophy, creatine is dramatically increased. Deficiencies in serum calcium, phosphorus, and magnesium may result in muscle cramping and spasms but do not represent the clinical picture described (Hoekelman, et al., p. 425; Huether & McCance, pp. 108, 484).

12. **(b)** Osgood-Schlatter's is a benign condition resulting from over use and is best treated with rest and supportive therapy (Burns, et al., p. 786).

13. **(a)** When there is no response to more conservative treatment interventions, such as passive stretching and environmental stimulation, surgery is the recommended course of action (Hoekelman, et al., p. 1139)

14. **(c)** Although still recommended in some sources, triple diapering is not thought to be effective because the musculoskeletal forces are greater than those exerted by diapers. Swaddling and the prone position are contraindicated and may increase the risk of dislocation (Burns, et al., pp. 780-781 Fox, p. 655).

15. **(d)** After the age of six months, both the Barlow and Ortolani maneuvers are less reliable due to diminished laxity in the hip. After two months soft tissue contractures may develop, making these tests unreliable (Fox, p. 631).

16. **(a)** Osteomyelitis is frequently associated with local trauma, whereas toxic synovitis is more commonly associated with a recent upper respiratory illness (Hoekelman, et al., pp. 944, 1469).

17. **(b)** Observing the patella can be very helpful in differentiating internal tibial

torsion from internal femoral torsion. The patella will rotate inward if the problem is above the knee. There is also general ligamentous laxity in other areas (fingers, elbows) associated with internal tibial torsion (Burns, et al., p. 787; Hoekelman, et al., p. 977).

18. **(c)** Metatarsus adductus is a flexural deformity of the foot related most commonly to intrauterine positioning. Flexible deformities, that is movement past the imaginary line extending from the middle of the heel through the second toe, can be managed with stretching exercises (Burns, et al., p. 788).

19. **(a)** This is the characteristic rash associated with systemic juvenile arthritis that occurs in 25% to 50% of children (Burns, et al., p. 508).

20. **(d)** The Adam's sign is demonstrated by having the child bend from the waist and observing for symmetry, and is part of the spinal examination to detect scoliosis. The Trendelenberg sign evaluates the stability of the muscles around the hip and is not diagnostic in scoliosis (Burns, et al., p. 774).

21. **(c)** "Little League" elbow or epicondylitis is a result of repetitive forearm supination and pronation. Therefore, the goal is to prevent the injury by reducing the repetitive motion. Ice falsely reassures parent or coach that the injury can be prevented by applying before and after pitching (Fox, p. 212).

References

Behrman, R. E., & Kliegman, R. M. (Eds.). (1998). *Nelson essentials of pediatrics* (3rd ed.). Philadelphia: W. B. Saunders.

Burns, C. E., Barber, N., Brady, M. A., & Dunn, A. M. (Eds.). (1996). *Pediatric primary care: A handbook for nurse practitioners.* Philadelphia: W. B. Saunders.

Fox, J. A. (Ed.). (1997). *Primary health care of children.* St. Louis: Mosby.

Hoekelman, R. A., Friedman, S. B., Nelson, N. M., Seidel, H. M., & Weitzman, M. L. (Eds.). (1997). *Primary pediatric care.* St. Louis: Mosby.

Huether, S. E., & McCance, K. L. (Eds.). (1996). *Understanding pathophysiology.* St. Louis: Mosby.

Note: This chapter was written by Patricia Clinton prior to her appointment as certification chair representing the National Association of Pediatric Nurse Associates and Practitioners (NAPNAP) to the National Certification Board of Pediatric Nurse Practitioners and Nurses.

Neurological Disorders

Martha K. Swartz

Select one best answer to the following questions.

1. A 5-month-old boy, a former 28-week-premature infant, is being evaluated in your practice because of a concern about delayed motor development. In formulating the differential diagnosis, you keep in mind that spastic cerebral palsy is characterized by:

   a. Increased deep tendon reflexes and sustained clonus
   b. Dystonic posturing
   c. Abnormal involuntary movements
   d. Nystagmus

2. A 4-year-old child with a history of myelomeningocele and a ventriculoperitoneal shunt presents to the clinic with a headache, nausea, vomiting, and lethargy. The most probable diagnosis is:

   a. Viral gastroenteritis
   b. Shunt malfunction
   c. Meningitis
   d. Shunt infection

3. An apparently healthy child, who is enrolled in Headstart, is suspected of having developmental delays based on Denver II results at two separate clinic visits. The most appropriate next step would be to:

   a. Request developmental evaluation from the Headstart program
   b. Repeat the Denver II in six months
   c. Refer the child for a more definitive evaluation
   d. Discuss ways in which parents can foster the child's development

4. Amanda is a 6-month-old infant recovering from a viral illness. At the peak of her illness (two days ago) she spiked a temperature of 104° F and experienced a febrile seizure. Amanda's mother is young and inexperienced, but is very

open to teaching. She wants to know if the seizure will "do anything" to Amanda. While teaching this new mother about simple febrile seizures, it would be accurate to say that Amanda:

    a. Is at increased risk for epilepsy as an adult
    b. Would benefit from phenytoin prophylaxis
    c. May experience repeated seizures
    d. Would benefit from phenobarbital prophylaxis

5. Which of the following signs is not characteristic of generalized seizures?

    a. Unilateral motor manifestations
    b. Disturbance of consciousness
    c. Tonic stiffening of the trunk
    d. Simultaneous and symmetric cerebral hemisphere discharge

6. Which of the following is the primary diagnostic tool used in the evaluation of seizure disorder?

    a. EEG
    b. Cerebral blood flow studies
    c. CT scan
    d. MRI

7. Upon physical examination of a 4-year-old boy you note seven café-au-lait spots greater than 5 mm in diameter. This finding may be indicative of:

    a. Tuberous sclerosis
    b. Sturge-Weber disease
    c. Duchenne's dystrophy
    d. Neurofibromatosis

8. Michael is a 15-year-old high school student who presents for a school sports physical. He appears to be in good health, but is concerned about a bad headache he had a few weeks ago. He is concerned becaue his mother's friend died of a brain tumor. You tell Michael that the most common type of headache with onset in adolescence is:

    a. Sinus headache
    b. Vascular headache
    c. Tension headache
    d. Migraine headache

9. An 18-year-old college freshman is seen in the student clinic with a complaint

of migraine headaches. In collecting the history, you keep in mind that migraine headaches are associated with:

a. Chronic, progressive pain
b. A positive family history   75%
c. Feelings of inadequacy or depression
d. Problems at home or school

10. Which of the following historical points would not alert the practitioner to the possibility of a brain tumor?

a. Headache in the morning associated with vomiting
b. A progressive headache worsening in frequency and severity
c. Deterioration in social, school, or athletic prowess
d. Chronic, recurrent headaches in an adolescent

11. Which of the following signs is not scored in the Glasgow Coma Scale?

a. Eye opening
b. Verbal response
c. Upper limb response
d. Fine motor response not scored

12. Mr. Harris calls the pediatric clinic to say that Josh, his 2-year-old son, has tripped on the sidewalk and hit his head on concrete. Which of the following symptoms reported by Mr. Harris would require that Josh be seen in the emergency room?

a. Uncontrollable crying no
b. Loss of consciousness
c. Scalp laceration no
d. History of febrile seizures no

13. A 2-year-old is evaluated in the emergency department for a closed head injury following a ten foot fall from an open window. When interpreting diagnostic imaging results, you are aware that the most common and generally the least serious type of skull fracture is:

a. Basilar fracture
b. Compound fracture
c. Depressed fracture
d. Linear fracture

14. A 12-month-old child, whose parents have a history of noncompliance for routine care, presents to the clinic with fever, irritability, and nuchal rigidity. The most critical diagnostic step in the child with suspected meningitis is:

    a. The history
    b. The physical examination
    c. Evaluation of the CSF
    d. Blood culture

15. In a child with suspected meningitis, the lumbar puncture should be delayed and a CT scan obtained first in which of the following circumstances?

    a. The child has altered pupillary responses $2°↑ ICP$
    b. The child has tachycardia
    c. The child has a negative Brudzinski sign
    d. The WBC is > 10,000/mm^3

16. Primary immunization is of paramount importance for preventing meningitis due to:

    a. *H. influenzae* type b ✓
    b. *N. meningitidis*
    c. *E. coli*
    d. *Klebsiella pneumoniae*

17. Kelly is a new mother trying to learn how to take good care of her 2-month-old infant. During the well-baby examination Kelly asks what Reye's syndrome is. She heard that it is very bad and she doesn't want her baby to get it. The PNP tells Kelly that to prevent the development of Reye's syndrome she should:

    a. Notify the PNP for a temperature > 100.4° F
    b. Be sure that their child receives the Varivax vaccine
    c. Avoid the use of aspirin in febrile illnesses
    d. Inquire about prophylactic therapy at the six month visit

18. The most common brain tumor of childhood is:

    a. Ependymoma
    b. Brain stem tumor
    c. Craniopharyngoma
    d. Astrocytoma

19. In most States, a learning disability is defined based on:

a. The child's IQ as determined by a psychological evaluation
b. A discrepancy between the child's actual and expected achievement
c. A diagnosis of attention deficits
d. Achievement test scores

20. Developmental dysgraphia refers to a learning disability characterized by disorders in:

a. Writing
b. Reading
c. Spelling
d. Mathematics

21. Which of the following is a measure of childhood intelligence?

a. Wechsler scales
b. Denver II   *development*
c. Bayley scales *development*
d. Vineland scales *adaptive behavior*

Answers & Rationale

1. **(a)** In spastic CP, a lowered reflex threshold results in increased DTRs and sustained clonus. The other signs are characteristic of dyskinetic and ataxic CP (Pellegrino, pp. 821-822).

2. **(b)** Headache, nausea, vomiting, and lethargy are frequently associated with malfunctioning shunt systems (Charney & Blum, p. 818).

3. **(c)** If a developmental lag is suspected based on repeated performances on the Denver II (which is a screening tool), a more definitive assessment should be obtained (Frankenburg, et al., p. 13).

4. **(c)** Children with a diagnosis of simple febrile seizures may experience repeated febrile seizures, particularly if the first seizure occurred before age one. They are not at increased risk for epilepsy as adults and phenytoin is not efficacious as a prophylactic drug, nor is phenobarbitol routinely recommended (Clancy, p. 705).

5. **(a)** In generalized seizures, motor manifestations, if any, are bilateral (Clancy, p. 702).

6. **(a)** In the study of seizure disorders, the EEG has the greatest clinical applicability. The other imaging techniques are considered supplemental (Moe & Seay, p. 635).

7. **(d)** More than six café-au-lait spots (greater than 5 mm in diameter) in prepubertal children is an essential part of the diagnosis of neurofibromatosis (Moe & Seay, p. 672).

8. **(c)** The most common headache in adolescents is the tension/psychogenic headache (Moe & Seay, p. 657).

9. **(b)** There is a positive family history in 75% of migraine headache cases. Progressive severity is associated with increased intracranial pressure or brain tumor. Emotional problems may be related to tension headaches (Moe & Seay, p. 657).

10. **(d)** The peak age range for brain tumors is age 3 to 10. Headache of recent onset is more worrisome (Moe & Seay, p. 657).

11. **(d)** The Glasgow Coma Scale is based on eye opening, verbal response and best upper limb response (Tecklenburg, p. 766).

12. **(b)** Emergency care should be sought following head trauma if the child is unresponsive (Tecklenburg, p. 767).

13. **(d)** The linear fracture is the most common and has little serious clinical implication unless it overlies a vascular channel or penetrates an air sinus (Tecklenburg, p. 768).

14. **(c)** Collection of the CSF is the most critical diagnostic step in the child with suspected meningitis based on the history and physical examination (St. Geme, p. 664).

15. **(a)** If elevated intracranial pressure is suspected, a CT scan should be obtained first to avoid the complication of cerebellar or uncal herniation (St. Geme, p. 664).

16. **(a)** Recommended primary immunization schedules include vaccines licensed for use against *H. influenzae* type b (St. Geme, p. 668).

17. **(c)** Reye's syndrome, a rare type of encephalopathy that is associated with varicella and other systemic viral infections, is more likely to occur if the child has received salicylates (Moe & Seay, p. 686).

18. **(d)** Astrocytomas, most of which are low grade, are the most common brain tumors of childhood (Albano, et al, p. 787).

19. **(b)** In most states, a learning disability means a discrepancy between the child's actual and expected achievement (Blum, p. 863).

20. **(a)** Dysgraphia refers to a learning disorder which affects writing ability (Camp & Kozleski, p. 99).

21. **(a)** The Wechsler scales measure intelligence, the Denver and Bayley measure development, and the Vineland measures adaptive behavior (Camp & Kozleski, p. 94).

References

Albano, E. A., Stork, L. O., Greffe, B. S., Odom, L. F., & Foreman, N. (1997). Neoplastic disease. In W. W. Hay, Jr., J. R. Groothuis, A. R. Hayward, & M. J. Levin (Eds.), *Current pediatric diagnosis and treatment* (13th ed., pp. 781-803). Stamford CT: Appleton & Lange.

Blum, N. T. (1997). Learning disabilities. In M. W. Schwartz, T. A. Curry, A. J. Sargent, N. J. Blum, & J. A. Fein (Eds.), *Pediatric primary care: A problem-oriented approach* (3rd ed., pp. 863-867). St. Louis: Mosby.

Camp, B. W., & Kozleski, E. B. (1997). Developmental disorders. In W. W. Hay, J. R. Groothuis, A. R. Hayward, & M. J. Levin (Eds.), *Current pediatric diagnosis and treatment* (13th ed., pp. 86-110). Stamford, CT: Appleton & Lange.

Charney, E. B., & Blum, N. J. (1997). Myelomeningocele. In M. W. Schwartz, T. A. Curry, A. J. Sargent, N. J. Blum, & J. A. Fein (Eds.), *Pediatric primary care: A problem-oriented approach* (3rd ed., pp. 809-821). St. Louis: Mosby.

Clancy, R. R. (1997). Seizure disorders. In M. W. Schwartz, T. A. Curry, A. J. Sargent, N. J. Blum, & J. A. Fein (Eds.), *Pediatric primary care: A problem-oriented approach* (3rd ed., pp. 701-711). St. Louis: Mosby.

Frankenburg, W. K., Dodds, J., Archer, P., Bresnick, B., Maschka, P., Edelman, N., & Shapiro, H. (1990). *Denver II screening manual.* Denver: Denver Developmental Materials.

Moe, P. G., & Seay, A. R. (1997). Neurologic and muscular disorders. In W. W. Hay, J. R. Groothuis, A. R. Hayward, & M. J. Levin. (Eds.), *Current pediatric diagnosis and treatment* (13th ed., pp. 631-703). Stamford, CT: Appleton & Lange.

Pellegrino, L. (1997). Cerebral palsy. In M. W. Schwartz, T. A. Curry, A. J. Sargent, N. J. Blum, & J. A. Fein (Eds.), *Pediatric primary care: A problem-oriented approach* (3rd ed., pp. 821-828). St. Louis: Mosby.

St. Geme, J. W. (1997). Bacterial meningitis. In M. W. Schwartz, T. A. Curry, A. J. Sargent, N. J. Blum, & J. A. Fein (Eds.), *Pediatric primary care: A problem-oriented approach* (3rd ed., pp. 663-669). St. Louis: Mosby.

Tecklenburg, F. W. (1997). Head trauma. In M. W. Schwartz, T. A. Curry, A. J. Sargent, N. J. Blum, & J. A. Fein (Eds.), *Pediatric primary care: A problem-oriented approach* (3rd ed., pp. 763-771). St. Louis: Mosby.

Genitourinary/Gynecological Disorders/Pregnancy and Birth

Martha K. Swartz

Select one best answer to the following questions.

Questions 1 and 2 refer to the following scenario.

A 10-year-old boy comes to your clinic for evaluation of a suspected urinary tract infection (UTI).

1. Which of the following signs would lead you to include diagnoses other than UTI in the differential?

    a. Increased frequency *UTI*
    b. Penile discharge *STD, balanitis*
    c. Costovertebral tenderness *UTI*
    d. Dysuria *UTI*

2. The culture indicates sensitivity to trimethoprim/sulfamethoxazole. The boy is treated with this antibiotic for 10 days. The most appropriate follow-up in this case would include:

    a. Obtaining a urinalysis in two weeks
    b. Instructing the parents that the child should return to clinic if symptoms persist
    c. Teaching parents home monitoring with nitrite sticks
    d. Referring the child for a renal ultrasound

3. The most important laboratory test to be performed when a UTI is suspected in a school age child is:

    a. A CBC with differential
    b. A urine dipstick
    c. A clean catch urine for U/A and C/S
    d. A voiding cystourethrogram (VCUG)

4. Jay is a 9-year-old boy followed by your practice. He has had no significant health problems by history, but his mother is very concerned because he is "wetting himself." As you begin your history and physical examination, you keep in mind that the most common type of enuresis in school age children is:

    a. Primary nocturnal enuresis *90%*
    b. Occasional daytime enuresis
    c. Secondary nocturnal enuresis
    d. Primary diurnal enuresis

5. Which of the following statements is not true with regard to primary nocturnal enuresis?

    a. There is often a positive family history of enuresis *T*
    b. It appears to be related to maturational delay *T*
    c. Some night time wetters stop wetting without any form of treatment *T*
    d. The incidence is higher in girls than in boys *F* *♂ > ♀*

6. For some enuretic children, a trial of imipramine at bedtime may be worthwhile. In these cases, parents should understand that:

    a. This drug is given intranasally
    b. Mental health treatment may also be necessary
    c. This drug should be used primarily for camping or overnight trips
    d. Satisfactory results are achieved in approximately 20% of children

70% effective but c relapse

7. While examining a 4-month-old boy, you are unable to palpate one of the testes. The next most appropriate step is to:

    a. Reassure the parents that this is a normal finding
    b. Refer the child to an endocrinologist
    c. Re-examine the baby in two months
    d. Refer the child to a urologist

surgery p 6 mos of age

8. Which of the following is not true with regard to hypospadias?

    a. The meatus is formed along the dorsum of the penis
    b. It is one of the most common penile abnormalities *T*
    c. Circumcision should be deferred *T*
    d. A referral for an endocrine evaluation may be indicated *T*

ventral surface

9. Upon examination of a 2-month-old boy, you notice a swelling in the right inguinal canal. Your differential diagnosis would not include:

a. Diastasis recti   *Abd.*
b. Hydrocele of the spermatic cord ✓
c. Inguinal hernia ✓
d. Lymphadenopathy ✓

Questions 10 and 11 refer to the following scenario.

A 12-year-old girl presents to your clinic with symptoms of vaginitis including odor, dysuria, frequency, and discomfort.

10. Which of the following causes of vaginitis is most likely due to sexual transmission?

    a. Candida   *(yeast)*
    b. Chlamydia   *STD*
    c. Pinworms   *(parasite)*
    d. Gardnerella   *(BV)*

11. Upon further history, physical examination, and laboratory screening, the girl is diagnosed with *Candida albicans* vaginitis. Appropriate treatment would include:

    a. Avoiding bubble baths   *vaginitis (NSp)*
    b. Topical acyclovir   *herpes*
    c. Ceftriaxone   *STD*
    d. Clotrimazole

12. A labial adhesion extending from the posterior fourchette to the clitoris is noted during the routine assessment of a 4-year-old girl. There is no history of difficulty voiding, dysuria, or discomfort. The most appropriate initial management is to:

    a. Recommend mechanical lysis using petrolatum ointment
    b. Prescribe a topical application of estrogen cream   *only if Sx*
    c. Refer to a GU specialist
    d. Reassure parents that no specific treatment is needed at this time

13. Patients with acute nephrotic syndrome may present with all but which of the following signs:

    a. Macroscopic hematuria
    b. Hypertension
    c. Oliguria
    d. Rebound abdominal tenderness

14. It is important to look for evidence of a preceding streptococcal infection when ruling out acute nephritis. This is best done by:

    a. Throat culture
    b. Skin examination
    c. ASO titer   ↑ in 80% of pts.
    d. ESR

15. When providing care for a preterm infant, you would be particularly concerned about:

    a. Meconium aspiration syndrome
    b. Retinopathy
    c. Pyloric stenosis
    d. Phenylketonuria

16. Which of the following is not characteristic of physiologic jaundice in a newborn?

    a. It occurs in about 59% of term newborns ✓
    b. The onset is within the first 24 hours of life   ⫽ 24° of age
    c. It is associated with bilirubin levels > 5 to 7 mg/dL ✓
    d. It may be due to inefficient hepatic function ✓

17. What is the primary pathophysiology of respiratory distress syndrome (RDS) in the neonate?

    a. Retained fetal lung fluid
    b. Infection
    c. Surfactant deficiency
    d. Overdistended alveoli

18. The most common abdominal mass in a neonate is:

    a. Wilm's tumor no
    b. Meckel's diverticulum no
    c. Neuroblastoma no – brain
    d. Renal dysplasia/hydronephrosis no - flank

19. An adolescent boy presents to the clinic with a painless mass in the left side of his scrotum. The most likely diagnosis is:

    a. Epididymitis
    b. Testicular torsion

c. Incarcerated hernia

d. Hydrocele

20. A foul smelling vaginal discharge that emits a fish odor when combined with 10% potassium hydroxide is most likely due to:

a. *Gardnerella vaginalis*   "BV"

b. *Candida albicans*

c. *Chlamydia trachomatis*

d. *N. gonorrhoeae*

21. A 17-year-old sexually active girl with chancres in the genital area is noted to have a positive Venereal Disease Research Laboratories (VDRL) test. The next step should be to:

a. Treat with ceftriaxone

b. Perform a specific treponemal antibody test   Syphilis

c. Culture for *C. trachomatis*

d. Discuss safer sex practices

22. The most common bacterial cause of a sexually transmitted disease (STD) is:

a. *Neisseria gonorrhoeae*

b. *Trichomonas vaginalis*

c. *Chlamydia trachomatis*

d. Herpes simplex

Answers & Rationale

1. **(b)** Classic signs of a UTI include enuresis, frequency, dysuria, urgency, fever and CVA tenderness. Discharge may indicate balanitis or a sexually transmitted disease (Lum, p. 629).

2. **(d)** Older boys with a first infection should be examined for urinary tract abnormalities. The other laboratory tests do not assess for urinary tract anomalies (Lum, p. 628).

3. **(c)** A clean catch midstream collection of urine is usually satisfactory to obtain a specimen for culture and sensitivity (Lum, p. 629).

4. **(a)** Ninety percent of enuretic children have primary nocturnal enuresis e.g., they are wet only at night during sleep and have never had a sustained period of dryness (Clark, p. 195).

5. **(d)** The incidence of primary nocturnal enuresis is three times higher in boys than in girls (Clark, p. 195).

6. **(c)** Imipramine is effective in about 70% of children. Because many patients relapse, however, its primary use is for camp or overnight visits (Clark, p. 196).

7. **(c)** If spontaneous descent of the testis does not occur, surgical correction should be done optimally between 6 and 12 months of age primarily to reduce the risk of infertility (Seidel & Gearhart, p. 1357).

8. **(a)** In hypospadias, the meatus opens on the ventral surface. In epispadias, which occurs less frequently, the opening is along the dorsal surface (Seidel & Gearhart, p. 1355).

9. **(a)** Diastasis recti is a midline fascial attenuation extending from the umbilicus to the xiphoid process (Cox & Zeigler, p. 429).

10. **(b)** Papillomas, trichomonas, herpes simplex, gonococcal, and chlamydial disease carry a high suspicion for sexual transmission. Candida typically occurs after a course of antibiotics, gardnerella is indigenous vaginal flora, and pinworms is a parasitic disease (Sigel, pp. 1095-1105).

11. **(d)** In *Candida albicans*, local application of clotrimazole, miconazole, and ticonazole appear to be equally effective (Schwarz, p. 684).

12. **(d)** If there is no evidence of UTI, obstruction, or discomfort, and parents are not unusually concerned, then no treatment is necessary. Estrogen cream may be initiated if treatment is urgently desired by the parents in spite of counseling. Spontaneous resolution usually occurs in a manner of months and is more effective than surgical or mechanical lysis (Howard, p. 1397).

13. **(d)** While pain in the abdomen or flank may be common in acute nephrotic syndrome, palpation of the abdomen usually reveals no significant findings (Ruley, p. 1436).

14. **(c)** The antistreptolysin O (ASO) titer is elevated in 80% of patients with a preceeding streptococcal infection (Ruley, p. 1437).

15. **(b)** Retinopathy is a problem associated with prematurity unlike meconium aspiration and pyloric stenosis. Phenylketonuria is an inborn error of metabolism (Philip, p. 135).

16. **(b)** In physiologic jaundice, clinical jaundice appears after 24 hours of age (Rosenberg & Thilo, p. 50).

17. **(c)** Respiratory distress syndrome or hyaline membrane disease is caused by a deficiency of surfactant which results in poor lung compliance and atelectasis (Rosenberg & Thilo, p. 44).

18. **(d)** Most abdominal masses are associated with the kidneys (multicystic/dysplastic or hydronephrosis) (Rosenberg & Thilo, p. 26).

19. **(d)** A hydrocele is not associated with pain while the other suggested diagnoses are (Cox & Ziegler, p. 430).

20. **(a)** Bacterial vaginosis, often caused by an overgrowth of *Gardnerella vaginosis,* is suspected on the basis of a malodorous vaginal discharge and positive "whiff" test when mixing the discharge with potassium hydroxide (Sigel, p. 1101).

21. **(b)** If the VDRL is positive, a specific treponemal test such as FTA-ABs should be done to confirm the diagnosis. Treatment is with benzathine penicillin G (Sigel, p. 1102).

22. **(c)** Chlamydia is the most common bacterial cause of STD with 4 million cases annually (Sigel, p. 1096).

References

Clark, R. B. (1997). Psychosocial aspects of pediatrics and psychiatric disorders. In W. W. Hay, Jr., J. R. Groothuis, A. R. Hayward, & M. J. Levin (Eds.), *Current pediatric diagnosis and treatment* (13th ed., pp. 177-209). Stamford, CT: Appleton & Lange.

Cox, J. A., & Ziegler, M. M. (1997). Lumps and bumps. In M. W. Schwartz, T. A. Curry, A. J. Sargent, N. J. Blum, & J. A. Fein (Eds.), *Pediatric primary care: A problem-oriented approach* (3rd ed., pp. 425-432). St. Louis: Mosby.

Howard, B. J. (1997). Labial adhesions. In R. A. Hoekelman, S. B. Friedman, N. M. Nelson, H. M. Seidel, & M. L. Weitzman (Eds.), *Primary pediatric care* (3rd ed., pp. 1396-1397). St. Louis: Mosby.

Lum, G. M. (1997). Kidney and urinary tract. In W. W. Hay, Jr., J. R. Groothuis, A. R. Hayward, & M. J. Levin (Eds.), *Current pediatric diagnosis and treatment* (13th ed., pp. 607-630). Stamford, CT: Appleton & Lange.

Philip, A. G. S. (1996). *Neonatology: A practical guide* (4th ed., pp. 163-169). Philadelphia: W. B. Saunders.

Rosenberg, A. A., & Thilo, E. H. (1997). The newborn infant. In W. W. Hay, Jr., J. R. Groothuis, A. R. Hayward, & M. J. Levin (Eds.), *Current pediatric diagnosis and treatment* (13th ed., pp. 20-76). Stamford, CT: Appleton & Lange.

Ruley, E. J. (1997). Nephritis. In R. A. Hoekelman, S. B. Friedman, N. M. Nelson, H. M. Seidel, & M. L. Weitzman (Eds.), *Primary pediatric care* (3rd ed., pp. 1435-1442). St. Louis: Mosby.

Schwarz, D. F. (1997). Sexually transmitted diseases. In M. W. Schwartz, T. A. Curry, A. J. Sargent, N. J. Blum, & J. A. Fein (Eds.), *Pediatric primary care: A problem-oriented approach* (3rd ed., pp. 681-691). St. Louis: Mosby.

Seidel, H. M., & Gearhart, J. P. (1997). Hypospadias, epispadias, and cryptorchism. In R. A. Hoekelman, S. B. Friedman, N. M. Nelson, H. M. Seidel, & M. L. Weitzman (Eds.), *Primary pediatric care* (3rd ed., pp. 1355-1357). St. Louis: Mosby.

Sigel, E. J. (1997). Sexually transmitted diseases. In W. W. Hay, J. R. Groothuis, A. R. Hayward, & M. J. Levin (Eds.), *Current pediatric diagnosis and treatment* (13th ed., pp. 1095-1105). Stamford, CT: Appleton & Lange.

Hematological Disorders

Brenda Holloway

Select one best answer to the following questions.

1. A 3-year-old male with known glucose-6-phosphate dehydrogenase (G-6-PD) deficiency has acute purulent otitis media. This child should not be treated with which of the following drugs?

    a. Amoxicillin
    b. Amoxicillin-clavulanate
    c. Erythromycin
    d. Trimethoprim/sulfamethoxazole   *sulfa*

2. Mrs. C. has brought her 2-year-old daughter, April, to the clinic with complaints of anorexia and irritability for the past several weeks. You note that she is afebrile and appears pale. Based on the signs and symptoms, which initial action is appropriate?

    a. Ask Mrs. C. to describe April's diet prior to her illness
    b. Prescribe supplemental iron therapy to be given three times a day
    c. Order laboratory work to assess red blood cell count and indices
    d. Refer April to a pediatrician for further evaluation

3. Mrs. B. has brought 5-year-old John to the clinic. She reports that he has been lethargic and has been running a low grade fever for about two weeks. Physical examination reveals no significant findings other than pallor and lymphadenopathy. A complete blood count reveals a decreased hematocrit, neutropenia, and thrombocytopenia. The practitioner's next action should be to:

    a. Prescribe a broad spectrum antibiotic and ferrous sulfate *no*
    b. Instruct Mrs. B. on the appropriate use of acetaminophen to treat John's fever *no*
    c. Reassure Mrs. B. that John's signs and symptoms are indicative of a viral infection *no*
    d. Refer John to a pediatrician for further evaluation

4. Routine laboratory studies have revealed that a 2-year-old has a decreased level of serum ferritin. Red cell count and indices are within normal limits for age. Based on this information, you may assume that the child:

   a. May have stage one iron deficiency anemia
   b. Likely has stage two iron deficiency anemia
   c. Likely has stage three iron deficiency anemia
   d. Does not have any stage of anemia

5. You have ordered a red blood count indices for a 10-year-old female. Results reveal a decrease in both the mean corpuscular hemoglobin (MCH) and the mean corpuscular volume (MCV). Differential diagnosis should include:

   a. Sickle cell anemia
   b. Vitamin B_{12} deficiency anemia
   c. Pernicious anemia
   d. Iron deficiency anemia

6. When planning screening protocols, it is important for the practitioner to know that iron deficiency anemia is most common in which life period(s)?

   a. The first month of life
   b. The period when the child is most sedentary
   c. The preschool years
   d. Periods of rapid growth

7. The PNP is teaching high school students about prevention of iron deficiency anemia. To teach prevention of the most common cause of iron deficiency in this age group, it is important to emphasize:

   a. Avoidance of all aspirin containing products
   b. A diet high in iron rich foods
   c. Avoidance of ingestion of carbonated beverages
   d. Avoidance of high fiber foods

8. You have prescribed iron supplements for a 3-year-old child. When instructing the mother how to give the iron preparation it is important to tell her that iron:

   a. Is best absorbed on an empty stomach
   b. Is best absorbed when given with meals
   c. Is best absorbed when given with milk
   d. Should not be given near bedtime

9. One month after prescribing iron therapy to treat iron deficiency in a child who has no other known health problems the PNP should:

   a. Teach the mother about iron rich foods
   b. Check the child's stools for occult blood
   c. Order a hemoglobin measurement
   d. Order a complete blood count

10. After treating a 2-year-old for iron deficiency anemia, laboratory tests show that his hemoglobin level has returned to normal. Which of the following actions is appropriate?

    a. Discontinue iron therapy and recheck his hemoglobin level in one month
    b. Discontinue iron therapy and tell the child's mother to reinitiate therapy if she notices any pallor
    c. Continue iron therapy until all the medicine at home is gone
    d. Continue iron therapy for two to three months *to build up Fe⁺ stores*

11. Baby Jason was born at 34 weeks gestation. He is now 10-weeks-old and his mother has brought him to your office for a routine examination. He appears alert and well developed. His mother tells you that he takes 2 to 4 ounces of formula every 2 to 4 hours around the clock. The plan for baby Jason should include which of the following?

    a. Initiation of rice cereal at bedtime
    b. Addition of two bottles of water each day
    c. Encouraging Jason's mother to limit his feedings to every 4 to 6 hours
    d. Prescribing ferrous sulfate to be administered three times a day

12. While evaluating the complete blood count (CBC) results of a 3-year-old child, the practitioner notes that in addition to hypochromia and microcytosis of the red cell, there are many poikilocytes and target cells. Based on this finding, differential diagnosis must include:

    a. Thalassemia major
    b. Iron deficiency anemia
    c. Pernicious anemia
    d. Vitamin B_{12} deficiency

13. When laboratory results reveal a hypochromic, microcytic anemia in a 2-year-old child, differential diagnosis must include:

    a. Lead poisoning
    b. Pernicious anemia

    c. Hemophilia

    d. Folic acid deficiency

14. The mother of a well developed, full term 3-week-old boy brings him to the clinic because he has been fussy and not eating well for the past week. A CBC reveals that he is anemic. When exploring the etiology of the anemia, it is important to know that which of the following is not a common cause of anemia in the newborn?

    a. Dietary iron deficiency

    b. Blood loss

    c. Hemolysis

    d. Decreased RBC production

15. To establish a diagnosis of sickle cell disease, which laboratory test is appropriate?

    a. CBC with RBC indices no

    b. Sickle cell prep no

    c. Sickledex no

    d. Hemoglobin electrophoresis

Questions 16, 17, and 18 refer to the following scenario.

Five year old Tonya has sickle cell disease.

16. To decrease the risk of vaso-occlusive crises, it is important to stress which of the following to Tonya and her parents?

    a. The need for frequent hand washing — ↓ infections

    b. The need for a diet high in iron

    c. Avoidance of the use of moth balls in the house

    d. Limitation of milk intake to one glass a day

17. Tonya's mother tells you that she is upset because Tonya sometimes wets the bed. A urinalysis reveals no significant findings. After review of the pathophysiology of sickle cell and vaso-occlusive crisis with her, which of the following should you tell the mother?

    a. To limit Tonya's fluids after dinner and especially at bedtime

    b. To keep reminding Tonya that most girls her age do not wet the bed

    c. To wake Tonya in the middle of the night and take her to the bathroom

d. To encourage Tonya to drink fluids and put a waterproof covering on her bed

18. Tonya's mother has brought her to the clinic because she has had fever of 101° F for the past two days and her appetite has been poor. Physical examination reveals no apparent cause for the fever. Appropriate treatment includes:

    a. Acetaminophen for fever and re-evaluating Tonya in 24 hours
    b. Ibuprofen for fever and re-evaluating Tonya in 24 hours
    c. Inpatient or outpatient antibiotic therapy
    d. No treatment unless the fever is above 102° F

19. To prevent complications of sickle cell disease during the ages 3 months to 5 years, daily doses of which medication should be prescribed prophylactically?

    a. Baby aspirin
    b. Acetaminophen
    c. Diphenhydramine
    d. Penicillin

20. Mrs. Sauls has brought her toddler to the clinic for an immunization update. While talking to her, you learn that they live in an old building that has been under renovation for the past two months. Based on this information, you should first assess the child for:

    a. Asbestosis
    b. Coccidioidomycosis
    c. Mold allergy
    d. Lead poisoning

Answers and Rationale

1. **(d)** Sulfa drugs precipitate hemolysis in patients with G-6-PD (Hoekelman, et al., p. 872).

2. **(a)** Anorexia and irritability usually indicate some illness or abnormality, and are common with anemia but are nonspecific. Pallor is associated with anemia but may also be caused by familial skin color, limited exposure to sun, vasoconstriction, and fear. Asking the mother about April's diet prior to illness will help determine whether April was receiving enough iron in the diet and help determine the differential diagnosis (Hoekelman, et al., p. 866).

3. **(d)** An abnormality of more than one formed element of the blood (RBC, WBC, or platelets) may indicate aplastic anemia (bone marrow dysfunction) or cancer, and should be evaluated by a physician (Hoekelman, et al., pp. 871, 1669).

4. **(a)** In the first stage of iron deficiency, the body's iron stores are decreased. This can be detected by a fall in serum ferritin. No red blood cell changes are present in the first stage of iron deficiency because there is enough iron to support red cell formation (Hoekelman, et al., p. 1377).

5. **(d)** Iron deficiency anemia is the most likely diagnosis of anemia characterized by microcytosis (decreased MCV) and hypochromia (decreased MCH) (Hoekelman, p. et al., 1379).

6. **(d)** The highest frequency of iron deficiency occurs during early childhood and adolescence, the same periods when growth is most rapid (Hoekelman, et al., p. 1376).

7. **(b)** Nutritional deficiency is the most common cause of iron deficiency anemia (Oski, et al., p. 1657).

8. **(a)** About twice as much iron is absorbed on an empty stomach as at mealtime. Iron is given with meals only if gastric irritation or nausea is a problem (Hoekelman, et al., p. 1379).

9. **(c)** When the child is otherwise healthy, recovery from iron deficiency anemia is about two thirds complete in one month. Re-evaluation of hemoglobin is recommended at one month. The mother should have already been taught about iron rich foods, and the stool would be checked initially or, now, only if positive response to iron therapy was not seen (Hoekelman, et al., p. 1379).

10. **(d)** After hemoglobin levels have been restored, additional iron supplements are needed to replete the body's iron stores (Hoekelman, et al., pp. 869, 1380).

11. **(d)** Because preterm infants have a smaller iron endowment and greater growth requirements after birth, oral iron supplements are recommended for preterm infants (Hoekelman, et al., p. 1376).

12. **(a)** Severe hypochromia and microcytosis as well as poikilocytes and target cells are seen in thalassemia. Poikilocytes and target cells do not characterize iron deficiency anemia. Pernicious anemia is macrocytic (Oski, et al., p. 1662).

13. **(a)** Lead poisoning causes hypochromic, microcytic anemia. Pernicious anemia and folic acid deficiency are associated with macrocytosis (Oski, et al., pp. 1658-1659).

14. **(a)** Iron deficiency caused by dietary deficiency is uncommon in the newborn. More common etiologies in this age are blood loss, hemolysis, and decreased red blood cell production (Hoekelman, et al., p. 873; Oski, et al., p. 1658).

15. **(d)** Sickle cell prep and sickledex are screening tests and do not differentiate between sickle cell trait and sickle cell disease. Diagnosis is dependent on hemoglobin electrophoresis (Fox, p. 153; Oski, et al., p. 1660; Hoekelman, et al., p. 873).

16. **(a)** Vaso-occlusive crisis is usually associated with infection, dehydration, acidosis, or exposure to cold. Many infections, especially respiratory, are largely spread by fomites, then hand to nose or eye contact (Hoekelman, et al., p. 873).

17. **(d)** Vaso-occlusive crisis is usually associated with infection, dehydration, acidosis or exposure to cold. Hemodilution helps prevent vaso-occlusion. Fluids should always be encouraged, and bed wetting is common in young children who drink fluids near bedtime (Hoekelman, et al., p. 873).

18. **(c)** If no simple cause is found for fever in patients with sickle cell disease, they should be treated as inpatients with IV antibiotics or outpatients with broad spectrum antibiotics (Hoekelman, et al., p. 873).

19. **(d)** Antibiotic prophylaxis is given to the child with sickle cell disease from ages 3 months to 5 years to reduce the risk of infection and subsequent vaso-occlusive crisis (Fox, p. 463).

20. **(d)** The main source of lead for children is dust in a house with deteriorated lead based paint. Any house built before 1960 is suspect, and renovation will result in airborne dust mixed with lead. Mold allergy is common but not as serious as lead poisoning. Answers ''a'' and ''b'' are uncommon in children compared to lead poisoning (Hoekelman, et al., p. 221).

References

Fox, J. A. (Ed.). (1997). *Primary health care of children.* St. Louis: Mosby.

Hoekelman, R. A., Friedman, S. B., Nelson, N. M., Seidel, H. M., & Weitzman, M. L. (Eds.). (1997). *Primary pediatric care* (3rd ed.). St. Louis: Mosby.

Oski, F. A., DeAngelis, C. D., Feigin, R. D., McMillan, J. A., & Warshaw, J. B. (Eds.). (1994). *Principles and practice of pediatrics.* Philadelphia: J. B. Lippincott.

Endocrine Disorders

Martha K. Swartz

Select one best answer to the following questions.

1. Screening for congenital hypothyroidism in newborns is accomplished by measuring:

   a. Thyroid stimulating hormone (TSH)
   b. Thyroxine (T_4) and TSH
   c. Triiodothyronine (T_3)
   d. T_4 binding globulin (TBG)

2. You are evaluating a 13-year-old girl for Grave's disease. Which of the following signs would not support this diagnosis?

   a. An enlarged thyroid
   b. Exophthalmos
   c. A positive family history
   d. An elevated TSH level   ↓TSH in Grave's Dz

3. The routine screening of a newborn in your practice indicates that the baby has congenital hypothyroidism and is in need of a referral to a pediatric endocrinologist. The treatment of choice for congenital or acquired hypothyroidism is:

   a. Levothyroxine
   b. Propylthiouracil
   c. Potassium iodide   } hyperthyroidism Rx
   d. Radiation therapy

4. A child in your clinic is being evaluated for short stature. Pertinent findings include delayed bone age, delayed onset of puberty and a stature that is normal for the child's bone age. The most likely cause of these findings is:

   a. Familial short stature
   b. Chromosomal abnormality

c. Constitutional delay of growth and development

d. Endocrine abnormality

5. Which chromosomal abnormality is associated with short stature in girls?

   a. Down syndrome
   b. Turner's syndrome
   c. Klinefelter's syndrome
   d. Prader-Willi syndrome

6. Achondroplasia refers to a growth delay that is:

   a. Due to malabsorption
   b. Associated with Noonan syndrome
   c. Associated with endocrine disorders
   d. Manifested by disproportionately short stature

7. You are following an infant girl in your practice with a history of breast development which appeared several months after birth and appears to be progressing. The PNP considers ordering a bone age, LH, FSH, and estradiol levels because she knows that most cases of premature telarche in girls are:

   a. A result of enzymatic defects
   b. Due to systemic CNS disease
   c. Idiopathic   80 % of girls
   d. A result of hypothyroidism

8. The mother of an 11-year-old boy is concerned that her son is developing secondary sexual characteristics too early. Your counseling for this family is based on the knowledge that puberty is considered precocious in boys if secondary sexual characteristics appear prior to age:

   a. 12
   b. 11
   c. 10
   d. 9

9. Treatment of true precocious puberty is best achieved with:

   a. Synthetic follicular stimulating hormone
   b. Gonadotropin releasing hormone
   c. Dexamethasone
   d. Thyroid hormone

10. The pathophysiology of type 1 diabetes is:

    a. Autoimmune destruction of the pancreatic beta cells
    b. Primary insulin receptor resistance
    c. Increased hepatic glucose production   *type II*
    d. Reduced glucose uptake by target tissue

11. An 11-year-old girl presents at a well child visit with symptoms of polyuria and polydipsia. Which of the following diagnoses must be ruled out?

    a. Diabetes mellitus
    b. Hyperthyroidism
    c. Adrenocortical insufficiency
    d. Nephrotic syndrome

12. For children with diabetes, in addition to home monitoring of blood glucose and urine ketone levels, glycosylated hemoglobin (Hgb A_{1c}) should be measured every:

    a. Week
    b. Month
    c. Three months
    d. Six months

13. Mrs. Williams has brought her 1-year-old baby to the clinic for a well baby examination. She is pregnant with her second child and is concerned about possible risks to the fetus because she has gestational class A diabetes. Which of the following conditions is the fetus not at risk for?

    a. Congenital anomalies
    b. Hypoglycemia
    c. Birth trauma
    d. Intrauterine growth retardation (IUGR)

14. Infants with IUGR are prone to hypoglycemia primarily because they:

    a. Have a decreased metabolic rate
    b. Have little carbon stores in the form of glycogen and fat
    c. Become acidotic
    d. Are prone to sepsis

15. During the first well baby examination of Joshua, a 2-week-old infant, his mother says that she is concerned because his penis is so small. Her sister has a friend whose baby had something called "ambiguous genitalia" and she is

afraid that Joshua has it too. When she asks if Joshua could get this condition, the PNP should tell her that the most common cause of ambiguous genitalia is:

  a. Idiopathic
  b. A chromosomal defect
  c. Congenital adrenal hyperplasia (CAH)
  d. An embryologic disorder

16. Which of the following signs or symptoms is not associated with congenital adrenal hyperplasia:

  a. Hypernatremia   ↓ Na, actually c̄ CAH
  b. Progressive weight loss
  c. Dehydration
  d. Hyperkalemia

17. Families of children with congenital adrenal hyperplasia should be educated about:

  a. The self-limiting aspect of the disorder
  b. The need for genetic counseling
  c. Dietary restrictions
  d. The need for chronic replacement therapy

18. A 14-year-old girl and her mother indicate to you that they are concerned because the girl has not yet started to menstruate. The history is noncontributory and the physical examination is normal. Breast development and pubic hair have been present for 12 months. The most appropriate initial step would be to:

  a. Do a pregnancy test
  b. Obtain a buccal smear for chromosomal analysis
  c. Reassure and educate the family
  d. Draw LH, FSH levels

19. Primary dysmenorrhea is due to:

  a. Elevated prostaglandin level
  b. Pelvic inflammatory disease (PID)
  c. Endometriosis   } Secondary dysmenorrhea
  d. Fibroids

20. The differential diagnosis of dysfunctional uterine bleeding includes all but which of the following:

    a. Pregnancy related disorders
    b. Anemia — *complication of DUB*
    c. Foreign body
    d. Endometriosis

Answers & Rationale

1. **(b)** CH screening is done prior to discharge and before day seven of life by measuring T_4 and TSH. If the T_4 is > 6.5 μg/dL and the TSH is >20 μU/mL, the infant should be referred to a pediatric endocrinologist (Fox, p. 758).

2. **(d)** In hyperthyroidism, the TSH level, which is under negative feedback control by the pituitary gland, is suppressed (Fox, p. 758).

3. **(a)** Levothyroxine is the drug of choice for treating hypothyroidism. Choices "b," "c," and "d" are treatments for hyperthyroidism (Fox, p. 758).

4. **(c)** Constitutional delay is characterized by a bone age that is delayed for chronological age and a normal growth velocity for bone age (Gruccio, p. 755).

5. **(b)** Turner syndrome, which occurs in girls, is associated with stature below the 3rd percentile in 99% of affected cases (Gruccio, p. 755).

6. **(d)** Achondroplasia, or skeletal dysplasia, is an autosomal dominant mutation that results in disproportionate short stature e.g., shortened limbs, macrocephaly, and bowing of legs (Gruccio, p. 753).

7. **(c)** Sexual precocity is idiopathic in 80% of girls (Weinzimer, et al., p. 539).

8. **(d)** Precocious puberty is defined as secondary sex characteristics appearing before age 9 in boys and age 8 in girls (Gotlin, et al., p. 844).

9. **(b)** Central precocious puberty is suppressible with analogues of long-acting gonadotropin-releasing hormone (GnRH) (Weinzimer, et al., pp. 539-540).

10. **(a)** Type 1 diabetes is an autoimmune disease in which islet cell antibodies destroy the pancreatic beta cells. The other causes of hyperglycemia are seen in type 2 diabetes (Kirchgessner, p. 858).

11. **(a)** Essential signs of diabetes mellitus include polyuria, polydipsia, weight loss, hyperglycemia, and glucosuria. Nephrotic syndrome may present following an influenza-like episode with periorbital swelling and oliguria (Kirchgessner, p. 858).

12. **(c)** HgbA$_{1c}$ should be measured every three months. This test reflects the frequency of elevated blood glucose levels over the previous three months (Chase & Eisenbarth, p. 861).

13. **(d)** The infant of a mother with gestational diabetes is often a macrosomic infant who is also at increased risk for trauma, congenital anomalies, and hypoglycemia (Rosenberg & Thilo, p. 65)

14. **(b)** IUGR infants have very little carbon stores in glycogen and body fat and therefore are prone to hypoglycemia (Rosenberg & Thilo, p. 65).

15. **(c)** CAH is the most common cause of ambiguous genitalia (Cheffer & Brady, p. 518).

16. **(a)** Hyponatremia (not hypernatremia) is a sign of CAH as there is excessive sodium loss through the kidneys and an inability to maintain serum electrolyte balance (Cheffer & Brady, p. 518).

17. **(d)** Families should be counseled about the need for lifelong medication therapy and follow-up (Cheffer & Brady, p. 519).

18. **(c)** Primary amenorrhea is defined by absence of menarche by 16 years of age with normal pubertal growth and development or absence of menarche two years after sexual maturation is completed. It is relatively uncommon and often due to constitutional delay (Barber, p. 723).

19. **(a)** Primary dysmenorrhea is due to an exaggerated production of uterine prostaglandins causing uterine hypercontractility, tissue ischemia, and nerve hypersensitivity. The other causes may lead to secondary dysmenorrhea (Barber, p. 725).

20. **(b)** Anemia is considered to be a complication of dysfunctional uterine bleeding rather than a part of the differential diagnosis (Barber, p. 727).

References

Barber, N. (1996). Gynecological conditions. In C. E. Burns, N. Barber, M. A. Brady, & A. M. Dunn (Eds.), *Pediatric primary care: A handbook for nurse practitioners* (pp. 717-735). Philadelphia: W. B. Saunders.

Chase H. P., & Eisenbarth, G. S. (1997). Diabetes mellitus. In W. W. Hay, Jr., J. R. Groothuis, A. R. Hayward, & M. J. Levin (Eds.), *Current pediatric diagnosis and treatment* (13th ed., pp. 857-863). Stamford, CT: Appleton & Lange.

Cheffer, N., & Brady, M. A. (1996). Endocrine and metabolic diseases. In C. E. Burns, N. Barber, M. A. Brady & A. M. Dunn (Eds.), *Pediatric primary care: A handbook for nurse practitioners* (pp. 513-528). Philadelphia: W.B. Saunders.

Fox, J. A. (1997). Thyroid disorders. In J. A. Fox (Ed.), *Primary health care of children* (pp. 756-759). St. Louis: Mosby.

Gruccio, D. (1997). Short stature. In J. A. Fox (Ed.), *Primary health care of children* (pp. 753-756). St. Louis: Mosby.

Gotlin, R. W., Kappy, M. S., & Slover, R. H. (1997) Endocrine disorders. In W. W. Hay, J. R. Groothuis, A. R. Hayward, & M. J. Levin (Eds.), *Current pediatric diagnosis and treatment* (13th ed., pp. 818-856). Stamford, CT: Appleton & Lange.

Kirchgessner, J. (1997). Diabetes mellitus. In J. Fox (Ed.), *Primary health care of children* (pp. 858-867). St. Louis: Mosby.

Rosenberg, A. A., & Thilo, E. H. (1997). The newborn infant. In W. W. Hay, J. R. Groothuis, A. R. Hayward, & M. J. Levin (Eds.), *Current pediatric diagnosis and treatment* (13th ed., pp. 20-76). Stamford, CT: Appleton & Lange.

Weinzimer, S. A., Lee, M. M., & Moshang, T. (1997). Endocrinology. In M. W. Schwartz, T. A. Curry, A. J. Sargent, N. J. Blum & J. A. Fein (Eds.), *Pediatric primary care: A problem-oriented approach* (3rd ed., pp. 529-541). St. Louis: Mosby.

Multisystem and Genetic Disorders

Patricia Clinton

Select one best answer to the following questions.

1. 17-year-old J.V. is diagnosed with *Neisseria gonorrhoeae*. Appropriate management would include treatment for which other sexually transmitted infection?

    a. Genital herpes
    b. Syphilis
    c. Chlamydia
    d. Trichomonas

2. Which of the following would be most helpful in confirming a diagnosis of nonspecific bacterial vaginosis?

    a. Gray discharge
    b. Fishy odor with KOH
    c. pH < 4.5
    d. Positive Fitz-Hugh-Curtis sign

3. T.L. is seen in student health and tests positive for syphilis. Which of the following interventions would be appropriate?

    a. VDRL titers at six weeks and three months
    b. Screen partners up to six months prior to infection
    c. Colposcopy examination of the cervix, vagina, and vulva
    d. Repeat clinical examination at three months and six months

4. R.C. is a 17-year-old female diagnosed with genital herpes and is receiving acyclovir. What patient education should you provide?

    a. Symptoms of vaginal candidiasis
    b. Use of topical acyclovir to reduce viral shedding *no*
    c. Use of condoms while lesions are present *no*
    d. Abstaining from sexual activity for 72 hours after beginning acyclovir *no*

5. Appropriate anticipatory guidance to decrease the risk of toxoplasmosis would include:

    a. When camping, treat water from streams with iodine
    b. Do not go barefoot in high risk areas
    c. Wash hands after changing cat litter
    d. Avoid handling contaminated diapers

6. Congenital toxoplasmosis and congenital cytomegalovirus (CMV) have similar clinical presentations. Which of the following is seen in cytomegalovirus but not in toxoplasmosis?

    a. Jaundice
    b. Microcephaly
    c. Cerebral calcifications
    d. Petechial rash

7. In the newborn examination of M.P., you hear a murmur suspicious for PDA and note an absent red reflex. The infant has also failed audiometric testing. This presentation is consistent with which of the following congenitally acquired disease?

    a. Cytomegalovirus
    b. Rubella
    c. Toxoplasmosis
    d. Group B streptococcus

8. 5-year-old L.T. is seen for a prekindergarten physical examination and immunizations. You learn that his father is HIV positive. Which vaccine should not be given?

    a. DTP
    b. MMR
    c. Oral polio   2° shedding of virus in stools
    d. DTaP

9. M.T. is HIV positive and has just delivered a 3.2 kg male infant. Which of the following should be included in her postpartum counseling?

    a. Suggest use of commercially prepared formula
    b. Encourage HIV testing of the infant at birth and at two months   no
    c. Avoid day care until infant has had two negative HIV tests   no
    d. Instruct that oral polio vaccine is contraindicated   no

10. You are examining S.K. in the newborn nursery. The prenatal history is significant for <u>alcohol abuse</u>. An important part of your <u>assessment</u> would be to:

    a. Observe for decreased bowel sounds
    b. Auscultate carefully for patent ductus
    c. Note passage of meconium
    (d.) Assess respiratory status carefully

    Trisomy 21 (DS)

11. During a newborn examination you observe <u>white specks</u> around the circumference of the iris. You would also want to assess <u>carefully</u> for which of the following?

    a. Hypertonicity
    b. Cherry red spot on macula
    (c.) Heart murmur   *DS*
    d. Cleft palate

12. Which of the following is associated with <u>Fragile X</u> syndrome but not with Turner's syndrome?

    (a.) Autism
    b. Delayed puberty
    c. Short stature
    d. Obesity

13. Which of the following ongoing assessments is of <u>low priority</u> in children with Turner's syndrome?

    a. Cardiac monitoring
    (b.) Vision screening
    c. Tanner staging
    d. Thyroid screening

14. You are part of a multidisciplinary team involved with the care of 13-month-old C.M. who has recently been diagnosed with <u>cerebral palsy, extrapyramidal type</u>. Which of the following statements is true with respect to C.M.'s type of cerebral palsy?

    a. Scoliosis is likely as the child grows
    b. Severe cognitive delays are expected
    c. The lower extremities are more likely to be involved
    (d.) It is associated with fewer seizures than CP with spastic quadriplegia

15. Appropriate management of a child with Klinefelter's syndrome would include replacement of which of the following?

    a. Thyroid hormone
    b. Growth hormone
    c. Estrogen
    d. Testosterone

16. S.G. is the 9-month-old child of Jewish parents seen for a routine well child examination. Mom states she seems more irritable lately and you note that she startles easily to noise. You should:

    a. Encourage mom to decrease environmental stimuli
    b. Refer to a pediatrician
    c. Refer for further developmental screening
    d. Re-evaluate at the 12 month examination

17. 16-year-year old D.S. is a tall, thin young woman who presents for a sports physical. She tells you she occasionally feels dizzy when sitting up, and sometimes has chest pain. You should be alert for a murmur associated with which of the following cardiac disorders?

    a. Mitral valve stenosis
    b. Pulmonic stenosis
    c. Aortic regurgitation
    d. Tricuspid regurgitation

18. 15-year-old M.C. appears acutely ill with a temperature of 102.5° F. Her period started three days ago. Physical examination is significant for a strawberry tongue and a scarlatinaform rash. The least helpful diagnostic test would be:

    a. BUN
    b. Rubella titers
    c. Rapid strep throat culture
    d. Urine creatinine

Answers and Rationale

1. **(c)** Chlamydia occurs in approximately 45% of gonorrhea cases and therefore it is recommended to treat both diseases (Burns, et al., p. 732; Hoekelman, et al., p. 1580).

2. **(b)** A gray discharge is associated with trichomoniasis and nonspecific bacterial vaginosis (NBV). A pH of < 4.5 suggests physiological leukorrhea rather than NBV which usually has a pH > 4.5. The Fitz-Hugh-Curtis sign indicates inflammation of the liver capsule seen in PID. The fishy odor after adding potassium hydroxide is a result of amines being released and is a classic of NBV (Behrman, et al., p. 249; Burns, et al., p. 732).

3. **(d)** Repeat clinical examinations and VDRL are recommended at three months and six months. Screening of partners prior to three months of onset of infection, and while symptomatic, is appropriate. Colposcopy examination is recommended for patients with evidence of HPV (AAP, p. 513; Burns, et al., pp. 730-732; Hoekelman, et al., p. 1588).

4. **(a)** Intercourse while active lesions are present should be avoided. Oral acyclovir is the treatment of choice for primary lesions (dose for seven to ten days) and/or recurrent lesions (dose for five days). Topical acyclovir does not decrease viral shedding. Candida infections are common sequelae in HSV infections (Burns, et al., p. 733; Hoekelman, et al., p. 1583).

5. **(c)** Transmission of toxoplasmosis occurs through handling of cat feces. Pregnant women should avoid contact with cat litter, and others should wash hands thoroughly when handling cat litter (Hoekelman, et al., p. 1492).

6. **(d)** A petechial rash is common in cytomegalovirus but rare in toxoplasmosis. Jaundice may be seen in both condions. Cerebral calcifications may also be found in both conditions. Microcephaly, which may appear at birth or manifest within a few months, is likewise seen in both CMV and toxoplasmosis (Burns, et al., p. 823; Katz, et al., p. 47).

7. **(b)** The classic presentation of congenitally acquired rubella includes intrauterine growth retardation, cataracts, microcephaly, and congenital heart disease

generally acquired during the first trimester (Katz, et al., p. 408; Burns, et al., p. 822).

8. **(c)** The oral polio vaccine should not be given because of viral shedding for several weeks following administration. DTP and DTaP are killed viruses and present no threat to others. Although MMR is a live virus, it does not shed and is therefore safe to administer (Burns, et al., p. 465).

9. **(a)** Human milk has been implicated in HIV transmission and therefore breast feeding should be avoided. Infants should be tested at one month and four months. There are no restrictions on day care. The regular immunization schedule should be followed. Infants who are HIV positive should receive IPV rather than OPV (APA, p. 281).

10. **(d)** FAS is associated with midfacial deformities including nasal deformities. Since infants are obligatory nose breathers, this may cause nasal obstruction and subsequent respiratory distress. ASD and VSD are the most common cardiac defects. Meconium stools are generally normal, as are bowel sounds (Fox, p. 952).

11. **(c)** White speckling of the iris is referred to as Brushfield spots which is associated with trisomy 21 syndrome (Down syndrome) but may also be a normal variant. Cardiac defects are common in trisomy 13 and require careful cardiac evaluation. Infants with trisomy 21 tend to be hypotonic rather than hypertonic. Cleft palate is associated with trisomy 13 (Fox, p. 52).

12. **(a)** Autism occurs in about 7% of males with Fragile X. Short stature and delayed puberty are characteristic of Turner's syndrome. Obesity is associated with Prader-Willi syndrome (Fox, pp. 53-54).

13. **(b)** Girls with Turner's syndrome are at risk for coarctation of the aorta, Hashimoto thyroiditis, and delayed appearance of secondary sexual characteristics (Zitelli & Davis, p. 272; Burns, et al., p. 860).

14. **(d)** CP with a spastic quadriplegia pattern often results in scoliosis, MR, and seizures. Atonic CP is associated with cognitive delays. The lower extremities are more often involved in spastic diplegia. Typically extrapyramidal CP has fewer seizures and less cognitive problems (Behrman, et al., p. 51).

15. **(d)** Klinefelter's occurs in males who exhibit tall slim bodies but inadequate virilization. The thyroid is not typically affected (Burns, et al., p. 235).

16. **(b)** Tay-Sachs's disease is seen in families of Ashkenazi Jewish descent, and is characterized by degenerative CNS signs and hyper-reaction to noise. Because of her ancestry, the possibility of Tay-Sachs should be explored (Behrman, et al., p. 730; Fox, pp. 43, 55).

17. **(a)** Individuals with Marfan's syndrome are tall and thin. Student athletes with this habitus should always be screened for cardiac problems including mitral valve stenosis. Mitral valve stenosis is characterized by chest pain, dizziness and syncope (Gartner & Zitelli, p. 165).

18. **(b)** The clinical presentation and history presented would suggest strep scarlet fever and toxic shock syndrome as differential diagnoses. A rapid strep screen would be easily obtained. With the history of menses, TSS is a serious and potentially life threatening possibility, and therefore a BUN and urine creatinine are warranted and easy to obtain. In TSS these are both significantly elevated. Fever and rash are present in rubella but the rash does not have the typical scarlatina presentation (Hoekelman, et al., pp. 1613-1617).

References

American Academy of Pediatrics (AAP). (1997). *Redbook: Report of the committee on infectious diseases* (24th ed.). Elk Grove Village, IL: Author.

Behrman, R. E., & Kliegman, R. M. (Ed.). (1998). *Nelson essentials of pediatrics* (3rd ed.). Philadelphia: W. B. Saunders.

Burns, C. E., Barber, N., Brady, M. A., & Dunn, A. M. (Eds.). (1996). *Pediatric primary care: A handbook for nurse practitioners.* Philadelphia: W. B. Saunders.

Fox, J. A. (Ed.). (1997). *Primary health care of children.* St. Louis: Mosby.

Gartner, J. C., & Zitelli, B. J. (Ed.). (1997). *Common and chronic symptoms in pediatrics.* St. Louis: Mosby.

Hoekelman, R. A., Friedman, S. B., Nelson, N. M., Seidel, H. M., & Weitzman, M. L. (Eds.). (1997). *Primary pediatric care.* (3rd ed.). St. Louis: Mosby.

Katz, S. L., Gershon, A. A., & Hotez, P. J. (Eds.). (1998). *Krugman's infectious diseases of children* (10th ed.). St. Louis: Mosby.

Zitelli, B. J., & Davis, H. W. (Eds.). (1997). *Atlas of pediatric physical diagnosis* (3rd ed.). St. Louis: Mosby.

Note: This chapter was written by Patricia Clinton prior to her appointment as certification chair representing the National Association of Pediatric Nurse Associates and Practitioners (NAPNAP) to the National Certification Board of Pediatric Nurse Practitioners and Nurses.

Health Policy

Martha K. Swartz

Select one best answer to the following questions.

1. Which of the following is true with regard to advanced practice licensure?
    a. It is granted by some States based on specialty certification
    b. It will guarantee reimbursement ⊢
    c. It may be obtained on a national basis ⊢
    d. It is a federal process verifying that a PNP has met standards for specialty practice ⊢

2. A PNP may obtain certification from the NCBPNP/N and the:
    a. American College of Nurse Practitioners
    b. American Academy of Nurse Practitioners
    c. American Nurses Credentialing Center
    d. American Nurses Association

3. The "Put Prevention into Practice" campaign to enhance the delivery of preventive care was initiated by the:
    a. Agency for Health Care Policy and Research
    b. U.S. Public Health Service
    c. NAPNAP
    d. Institute of Medicine

4. Payment by capitation means that:
    a. Financial risk is shifted from payers to providers
    b. Care is provided on a fee for service basis
    c. Care resources are rationed
    d. Target populations have unlimited access to health care

5. Managed care plans may be certified by the:

   a. Health Care Financing Administration (HCFA)
   b. Department of Health and Human Services (DHHS)
   c. National Institutes of Health (NIH)
   d. National Committee for Quality Assurance (NCQA) = HEDIS

6. Prescriptive writing privileges:

   a. Require a formal collaborative relationship with a physician
   b. Are regulated by both Boards of Nursing and Medicine
   c. Vary according to State statutes
   d. Are granted upon certification

7. Decreasing the fragmentation of clinical services is considered to be an integral part of:

   a. Prevention
   b. Case management
   c. Cost containment
   d. Health promotion

8. A main goal of continuous quality improvement is to:

   a. Incorporate norms, criteria, and standards as evaluative measures
   b. Emphasize outcome measures in addition to structure and process
   c. Promote evaluation based on peer review, audits, and chart reviews
   d. Inform that quality assurance is more than a periodic evaluation of performance

9. In documenting quality care, patient satisfaction is considered to be what type of measure?

   a. Structural
   b. Process
   c. Outcome
   d. Cost containment

10. Political activism through lobbying is an example of what type of change strategy?

   a. Normative re-educative
   b. Empirical rational
   c. Power-coercive = lobbying

d. Confrontational

11. The Early and Periodic Screening, Diagnostic and Treatment (EPSDT) program describes a comprehensive set of health care services as provided by:

a. Private insurance
b. State child protection teams
c. Medicaid
d. Most managed care organizations

12. Scope of practice statements:

a. Are prepared by national professional organizations
b. Provide the basis for reimbursement policies
c. Are written by employers
d. May vary from State to State

Answers & Rationale

1. **(a)** Licensure for advanced practice is available in many states if the applicant has demonstrated specialty certification (Porcher, p. 181).

2. **(c)** The American Nurses Credentialing Center (ANCC) and the National Certification Board of Pediatric Nurse Practitioners/Nurses (NCBPNP/N) are certifying bodies for a PNP (Porcher, p. 183).

3. **(b)** The USPHS initiated the Put Prevention into Practice (PPIP) program (Hickey, p. 14).

4. **(a)** In capitation, providers are responsible for a target population for which they receive an age and gender adjusted budget (Satinsky, p. 132).

5. **(d)** The NCQA certifies managed care plans utilizing a set of performance measures known as Health Plan Employer Data and Information Sets (HEDIS) (Cohen & Juszczak, p. 8)

6. **(c)** The extent of prescription writing privileges vary from State to State (Hawkins & Thibodeau, p. 86).

7. **(b)** Case management is an aspect of practice which provides quality, community based care while decreasing fragmentation of services (Cohen & Juszczak, p. 9).

8. **(d)** Continuous quality improvement is considered to be an integral (not just periodic) part of the organization (Hawkins & Thibodeau, p. 110).

9. **(c)** Outcome measures reflect the effects of care on health status, patient knowledge and satisfaction. Structural measures of care include the physical and organizational properties of the site, and process measures reflect what is actually done in giving and receiving care (Cohen & Juszczak, p. 8).

10. **(c)** Political activism through lobbying at local, state and national levels is an

example of coercive change strategies. The power of our vote will influence the actions of policy makers who represent us (Hawkins & Thibodeau, p. 75).

11. **(c)** EPSDT is intended to provide comprehensive care to Medicaid eligible individuals up to age 21 (Cohen & Juszczak, p. 4).

12. **(a)** Scope of practice statements are prepared by national professional organizations and may go beyond what is legally allowable in a given State (Hawkins & Thibodeau, p. 29).

References

Cohen, S. S., & Juszczak, L. (1997). Promoting the nurse practitioner role in managed care. *Journal of Pediatric Health Care, 11*(1), 3-11.

Hawkins, J. W., & Thibodeau, J. A. (1996). *The advanced practitioner: Current practice issues* (4th ed.). New York: Tiresias Press.

Hickey, J. V. (1996). Reformation of health care and implications for advanced nursing practice. In J. V. Hickey, R. M. Ouimette, & S. L.Venegoni (Eds.)., *Advanced practice nursing: Changing roles and clinical applications* (pp. 3-21). Philadelphia: J. B. Lippincott.

Porcher, F. K. (1996). Licensure, certification and credentialing. In J. V. Hickey, R. M. Ouimette, & S. L.Venegoni (Eds.), *Advanced practice nursing: Changing roles and clinical applications* (pp. 179-187). Philadelphia: J. B. Lippincott.

Satinsky, M. (1996). Advanced practice nurse in a managed care environment. In J. V. Hickey, R. M. Ouimette, & S. L.Venegoni (Eds.), *Advanced practice nursing: Changing roles and clinical applications* (pp. 126-145). Philadelphia: J. B. Lippincott.

Health Leadership Associates
Nurse Practitioner Continuing Education Programs

Analysis of the 12-lead ECG

This course is designed for advanced practice nurses. During this 8 hour course you will review cardiac electrophysiology, the cardiac cycle and cardiac muscle function as a basis for 12-lead ECG interpretation; analysis of dysrhythmia, conduction abnormalities, atrial abnormalities, ventricular hypertrophy, axis deviation, myocardial ischemia and myocardial infarction. A one hour practice workshop completes the program. A comprehensive course syllabus is included.

Pharmacology for Nurse Practitioners: A Comprehensive Review and Update

This 30 hour course is designed as a comprehensive presentation and review of pharmacology from the physiologic perspective. In addition to presenting the pharmacokinetics and pharmacodynamics of drugs (indications, contraindications, mechanisms of action, excretion and side effects profile) the corresponding body system physiology will be presented in a format that makes the pharmacology easy to understand and apply in clinical practice. A comprehensive course syllabus is included.

Suturing Review and Practice

This $2\frac{1}{2}$ hour course is designed for nurse practitioners who do not have significant suturing experience. Whether you have been taught but haven't practiced, or have never been taught at all, this program will introduce and reinforce skills that you have not had the opportunity to develop. A brief didactic session on wound assessment and preparation is followed by hands-on instruction and practice of the simple interrupted and vertical mattress techniques.

For information on these and other programs contact:
Health Leadership Associates, Inc.
P.O. Box 59153
Potomac, MD 20859
1-800-435-4775

For information on Certification Review Courses, Home Study Programs and Review Books contact:

Health Leadership Associates, Inc.
Post Office Box 59153
Potomac, Maryland 20859

1-800-435-4775

REVIEW BOOK/AUDIO CASSETTE ORDER FORM
HEALTH LEADERSHIP ASSOCIATES, INC.

PLEASE PRINT OR TYPE

NAME: _____

ADDRESS: Street _____ Apt. # _____ City _____ State _____ Zip Code_____

TELEPHONE: _____ (HOME) _____ (WORK)

Section 1: AUDIO CASSETTES

Professional "live" audio recordings of Review Courses are approximately 15 hours in length unless otherwise noted and include detailed course handouts. Continuing Education contact hours are available for these audio cassette Home Study Programs.

QTY	REVIEW COURSE TITLE	PRICE	
___	Acute Care Nurse Practitioner	$150.00	_____
___	Adult Nurse Practitioner	$150.00	_____
___	Analysis of the 12-Lead ECG (Available 6/99)	$75.00	_____
___	** Childbearing Management	$45.00	_____
___	Clinical Specialist in Adult Psychiatric and Mental Health Nursing	$150.00	_____
___	Family Nurse Practitioner (Consists of ANP, PNP & Childbearing Management Courses)	$330.00	_____
___	* Gerontological Nurse	$75.00	_____
___	Gerontological Nurse Practitioner	$150.00	_____
___	Home Health Nurse	$150.00	_____
___	Inpatient Obstetric/Maternal Newborn/ Low Risk Neonatal/Perinatal Nurse	$150.00	_____
___	Medical-Surgical Nurse	$150.00	_____
___	** Menopause Lecture	$30.00	_____
___	Midwifery Review	$150.00	_____
___	* Pediatric Nurse	$75.00	_____
___	Pediatric Nurse Practitioner	$150.00	_____
___	Pharmacology Review and Update (Available 4/99)	$300.00	_____
___	* Psychiatric and Mental Health Nurse	$75.00	_____
___	** Test Taking Strategies and Techniques	$20.00	_____
___	Women's Health Care Nurse Practitioner	$150.00	_____

* 8 Hour Course, ** 2 Hour Course

SUB TOTAL:		_____
Maryland Residents add 5% sales tax:		_____
CEU FEE ($25/course, except FNP course $35):	OPTIONAL	_____
Shipping: 2 Hour Course	$5.00	_____
All other Courses	$10.00	_____
TOTAL:		_____

PAYMENT DUE   METHOD OF PAYMENT

☐ Check or money order (US funds, payable to Health Leadership Associates, Inc.) A $25 fee will be charged on returned checks.

☐ Purchase Order is attached. P.O. # _____

☐ Please charge my: ☐ MasterCard ☐ Visa ☐ AMEX ☐ Discover

Credit Card# _____ Exp. date _____

Signature _____

Print Name _____

REVIEW GUIDES & AUDIO CASSETTES

1) Section 1 Total	$ _____	
2) Section 2 Total	$ _____	
3) Section 3 Total	$ _____	(All prices subject to change without notice)
TOTAL PAYMENT DUE	$ _____	

Section 2: REVIEW BOOKS

QTY	BOOK TITLE	PRICE	
___	Adult Nurse Practitioner Certification Review Guide (third edition)	$47.75	_____
___	Family Nurse Practitioner Certification Review Guide Set (Includes ANP, PNP, and Women's Health Care NP Guides)	$123.25	_____
___	Gerontological Nursing Certification Review Guide for the Generalist, Clinical Specialist, and Nurse Practitioner (revised edition)	$47.75	_____
___	Pediatric Nurse Practitioner Certification Review Guide (third edition)	$47.75	_____
___	Psychiatric Certification Review Guide for the Generalist and Clinical Specialist in Adult, Child, and Adolescent Psychiatric and Mental Health Nursing (second edition)	$47.75	_____
___	Women's Health Care Nurse Practitioner Certification Review Guide	$47.75	_____
___	TODAY and TOMORROW'S WOMAN – MENOPAUSE: BEFORE AND AFTER (Girls of 16 to Women of 99)	$10.00	_____

STUDY QUESTION BOOKS

QTY	BOOK TITLE	PRICE	
___	Acute Care Nurse Practitioner Certification Study Question Book	$30.00	_____
___	Adult Nurse Practitioner Certification Study Question Book	$30.00	_____
___	Family Nurse Practitioner Certification Study Question Book Set (Includes ANP, PNP and WHNP Study Question Books)	$60.00	_____
___	Pediatric Nurse Practitioner Certification Study Question Book	$30.00	_____
___	Women's Health Nurse Practitioner Certification Study Question Book	$30.00	_____

SUB TOTAL:		_____
Maryland Residents add 5% sales tax:		_____
CEU FEE ($20 per book, except FNP Set $35):	OPTIONAL	_____
Shipping: $9.00 FNP Set:		_____
$5.00 for one book:		_____
$2.00 for each additional book: (Except $1.00 for each add'l. Today and Tomorrow's Woman)		_____
TOTAL:		_____

For orders of 10 or greater call 1-800-435-4775.

Section 3: REVIEW BOOK/AUDIO CASSETTE DISCOUNT PACKAGES

A discounted rate is available when purchasing Review Book(s) and Audio Cassettes together. When purchasing packages, indicate Book/Audio Cassette selections in sections 1 and 2. *Does not apply to Study Question Books.* Calculate amount due in this section.

QTY	PACKAGE SELECTION	PRICE	
_____	8 Hour Course / 1 Review Guide	$120.00	_____
_____	15 Hour Course / 1 Review Guide	$190.00	_____
_____	FNP Package	$415.00	_____

FNP Package consists of Adult NP, Pediatric NP, Women's Health Care Guides & Audio Cassettes of the ANP, PNP, and Childbearing Management Courses.

SUB TOTAL:		_____
Maryland Residents add 5% sales tax:		_____
CEU Fee ($35 per package, except FNP Package $45)	OPTIONAL	_____
TOTAL: (Shipping charge included in package rate)		_____

RETURN POLICY

Due to the nature of the material contained in the review books and audio cassettes, returns on books ONLY will be accepted one week post delivery. No returns on audio cassettes except for defective audio cassettes which will be replaced.

MAIL TO:	Health Leadership Associates, Inc. P.O. Box 59153 Potomac, MD 20859
OR PHONE:	(800) 435-4775; (301) 983-2405
OR FAX:	(301) 983-2693

12/98

NOTES

NOTES

NOTES

NOTES

NOTES

NOTES

NOTES

NOTES

NOTES

NOTES

NOTES

NOTES

NOTES

NOTES

NOTES

NOTES

NOTES

NOTES